In The Eyes of an Alzheimer's Patient

By Gene Damm

Leaning Rock Press
Gales Ferry, CT

Copyright © 2022, Gene Damm

All rights reserved. No parts of this publication may be reproduced, stored in a database or retrieval system, or transmitted, in any form or by any means, without the prior permission of the author or publisher, except by a reviewer who may quote brief passages in a review.

Leaning Rock Press, LLC
Gales Ferry, CT 06335
leaningrockpress@gmail.com
www.leaningrockpress.com

Portrait of Mary on back cover by Christopher Morris

978-1-950323-74-6, Hardcover
978-1-950323-75-3, Softcover
978-1-950323-76-0, eBook

Library of Congress Control Number: 2022901538

Publisher's Cataloging-In-Publication Data
(Prepared by The Donohue Group, Inc.)

Names: Damm, Gene, 1934- author.
Title: In the eyes of an Alzheimer's patient / by Gene Damm.
Description: Gales Ferry, CT : Leaning Rock Press, [2022] | Includes bibliographical references.
Identifiers: ISBN 9781950323746 (hardcover) | ISBN 9781950323753 (softcover) | ISBN 9781950323760 (ebook)
Subjects: LCSH: Damm, Mary, 1935-2020. | Alzheimer's disease--Patients--Biography. | Alzheimer's disease--Patients--Family relationships. | Caregivers--Mental health. | LCGFT: Biographies.
Classification: LCC RC523.2 .H36 2022 (print) | LCC RC523.2 (ebook) DDC 362.1968310092--dc23

Printed in the United States of America

Dedication

This book is dedicated to my wife Mary
and to the many patients who are suffering from Alzheimer's,
as well as their caregivers,
who tirelessly take loving care of their patients.

Contents

I	Prologue
IV	The Seven Stages of Alzheimer's Disease
1	The Story Begins
10	The Beginning of Our Adventures Together
17	Our Early Life Together
22	Our Family Life and Gene's Career
43	Some of Our Travels
48	A Difficult Decision
53	Our Coaching Careers
61	Another New Adventure
66	A Major Change in the Road
71	Life at the Cottage
79	Starting a New Swimming Program
85	A Bump in the Road
91	A Major Bump in the Road
101	The Wall Starts to Crumble
119	The Beginning of the End
123	The Further Crumbling
126	And Then Came Martha
131	The Beginning of the Final Stages
133	Reality is Faced
138	My Final Days
147	The Plight of Others
169	A Note From the Author
178	A Few Words about Alzheimer's
188	Acknowledgments
189	Resources
190	References
191	Other Books by Gene Damm

Prologue

This book is dedicated to my wife Mary, and the many people who have suffered with the terrible disease of Alzheimer's. I am listed as the author, but I wrote most of this book in the eyes of an Alzheimer victim, using Mary as the patient. While the words are mine, I used her as the source. She had a knack for teasing without offending people, and I used some expressions typical of her in telling our story.

A few books have been written on Alzheimer's describing the path of the victim. Very few, if any, focus on the caregiver. This book focuses on both, but mainly on the caregiver's life before and after the Alzheimer's diagnosis. It describes how a wife changed the life of her husband from a follower to a leader, and eventually introduced him to a career helping others. It is a story of unending love, demonstrating that the victim and the caregiver can both suffer, sometimes with life ending consequences for the caregiver, as well.

While there is no cure for Alzheimer's, there are life controllable issues in the case of the caregiver, especially if the caregiver is a male unaccustomed to serving the combined role of cook, housekeeper, nurse, and valet all rolled into one. If you never, or seldom changed diapers, the transition can be dramatic, as well as exhausting. That is not taking away from the terrible life changes in the victim, and I feel bad about even emphasizing the caregiver so much, but it is a reality that is seldom discussed in novels, which is what most of us read. If the burden on the caregiver takes their life away from them, who is going to take care of the one they loved so dearly? Their story needs to be told as well.

Mary inspired me in many ways. I still feel her inspiration in telling our story from being relatively poor children to gaining recognition in a field, which had started out as volunteer activities. She was also a major reason for my success at IBM, by leading me to a more outgoing personality. She was the person who encouraged me to coach swimming and remain in it after some health issues. Coaching turned out to be my real love, as well as hers, as the hobby of coaching swimmers became a second career for me, and a career for her. It was a source of much enjoyment for both of us.

We were not perfect people, and certainly I am not a perfect man. I will point to many of our accomplishments, as well as some of our deficiencies in this book. Many people who think they know us well are still not aware of them. However, with apologies to you, the reader, I will not point out all our deficiencies.

We did not become well known multimillionaires, so it is not a rags to unbelievable riches story. It is a story of two people who meshed together in their zeal to help others. When we first volunteered as swimming coaches, we were able to afford the expenses of hotels and restaurants associated with coaching at away meets, because of my full-time job at IBM. Much of our life story shows how we climbed the wall of happiness, before we encountered the biological villain that attacked Mary's body. Mary helped me overcome a part of my subservient personality and be able to lead when I needed to. In the end I was able to control what I wanted to be. I had a rare combination of ego and inferiority complexes.

The coaching of swimmers became the only job for Mary and me when I retired from IBM at age 57, after my first heart attack. It was a never regretted decision that we both made together, as we usually did in our marriage. Mary was the leader in many of our decisions in our personal life.

A example of Mary leadership was when our team started to become a powerhouse in our local community. She boldly exclaimed, "If you want to be the best, then you swim (against) the best." This led to our going far beyond our local area and becoming a better team and coaches for it.

The key for us in our swimming/coaching career was that we were always together as a team. Most coaches do not have that luxury. Leaving their spouses and family home over long weekends is not good for family life, especially if their spouse had never experienced a swimming career. We also knew each other's flaws, and would fill the gaps. I was the technician, which was a role I loved, and Mary was my assistant coach, and record keeper, while preparing meet entries, a role I did not relish. I was the head coach, and she was the assistant coach. I was the analyst, and she was the details person. She loved doing that, and it would have been difficult for me to handle while working a full-time job. Besides, coaching was my love, not paperwork. While I was successful, as things go, in my job at IBM, coaching allowed me to fulfill the love of mine for teaching others. Besides swimmers, and assistant coaches, teaching my employees was my management style when I worked for IBM, but it was amplified in the coaching profession which Mary and I truly loved.

Within our Alzheimer's story, is woven the joy that comes from working together with young people and playing a role in their development. I hope this theme encourages others to do the same, even though, working all the long hours that we worked may not be good for their health and marriage. It should really be a balance situation, always keeping priorities straight.

The Seven Stages of Alzheimer's Disease[1]

Stage 1 is difficult to detect except through a chemical analysis of the brain. The patient of better than average intelligence may show very few signs of what is to come until more significant damage is done to the brain. They may even do well on some memory tests, but the chemicals that cause this dreaded and life ending disease may still be starting to show its power in the assault on the person's brain, as the disease diminishes their full capacity. It is interesting to note that a recent study by Arizona State University Edison college of Nursing and Health Innovation indicated that aerobic intervention significantly reduced the cognitive decline for patients with Alzheimer's dementia. In other words, while Alzheimer's typically progresses over a four to eight year timespan, a person who exercises regularly may be able to considerably expand that range.

In **Stage 2** it may still not be detected, and any memory recall may be associated in an observers mind with normal aging. It must be emphasized that the intervention must be done at this stage where the Alzheimer's patients are well enough, as well as mentally able to mobilize themselves before more deterioration takes place. As is the case in many diseases, early diagnosis and treatment help. Because Alzheimer's is very difficult to detect, even by medical professionals without expert testing, the window of diagnosis to lengthen the mental acuity and life of the patient can be shorter than you would like, before they reach the next critical stage.

In **Stage 3** the symptoms start to show in planning and organizing. The patient loses objects and cannot remember names and places. Does this sound like many an aging person? Even from a doctor's perspective, it may be confused with vascular dementia during the middle stages.

In **Stage 4** the patient may not remember dates and display difficulty ordering from a menu. It becomes difficult for them to drive a car in a safe manner. We were told, as an example, not to have Mary go near a stove or try to cook even in the very early stages. The hospital sensed that something was not right and was trying to figure out why she blacked out.

Stage 5 exhibits itself in significant confusion. The patient may need help in dressing and bathing properly, as well as eating. The challenge for the caregiver has begun. The patient may typically ask the same question over and over again. They still may remember the past, but it may be sketchy.

In **Stage 6** the patient shows confusion when asked questions, may be unaware of their surroundings, and in some cases have hallucinations, along with extreme personality changes. The difficult part for any caregiver is that they may not be able to control their bladder or bowel functions. Thus, a lot of support is involved in changing clothing, cleanup of the person and the house. This is the stage which challenges the caregiver, both physically and mentally.

In **Stage 7** the patient loses their ability to swallow as well as the ability to recognize that they are hungry or thirsty. It is the stage in which they will take their final breath. This is when the tragedy becomes total reality as the loved ones just have to sit and wait for the eventuality. No one can actually predict when the end will come. You just have to wait until the last breath is taken. The loved ones who had hoped that a recovery may have been possible as it had happened in earlier dire situations, now have to face facts. Family support for both the caregiver and the patient is critical at this stage.

*In The Eyes
of an
Alzheimer's Patient*

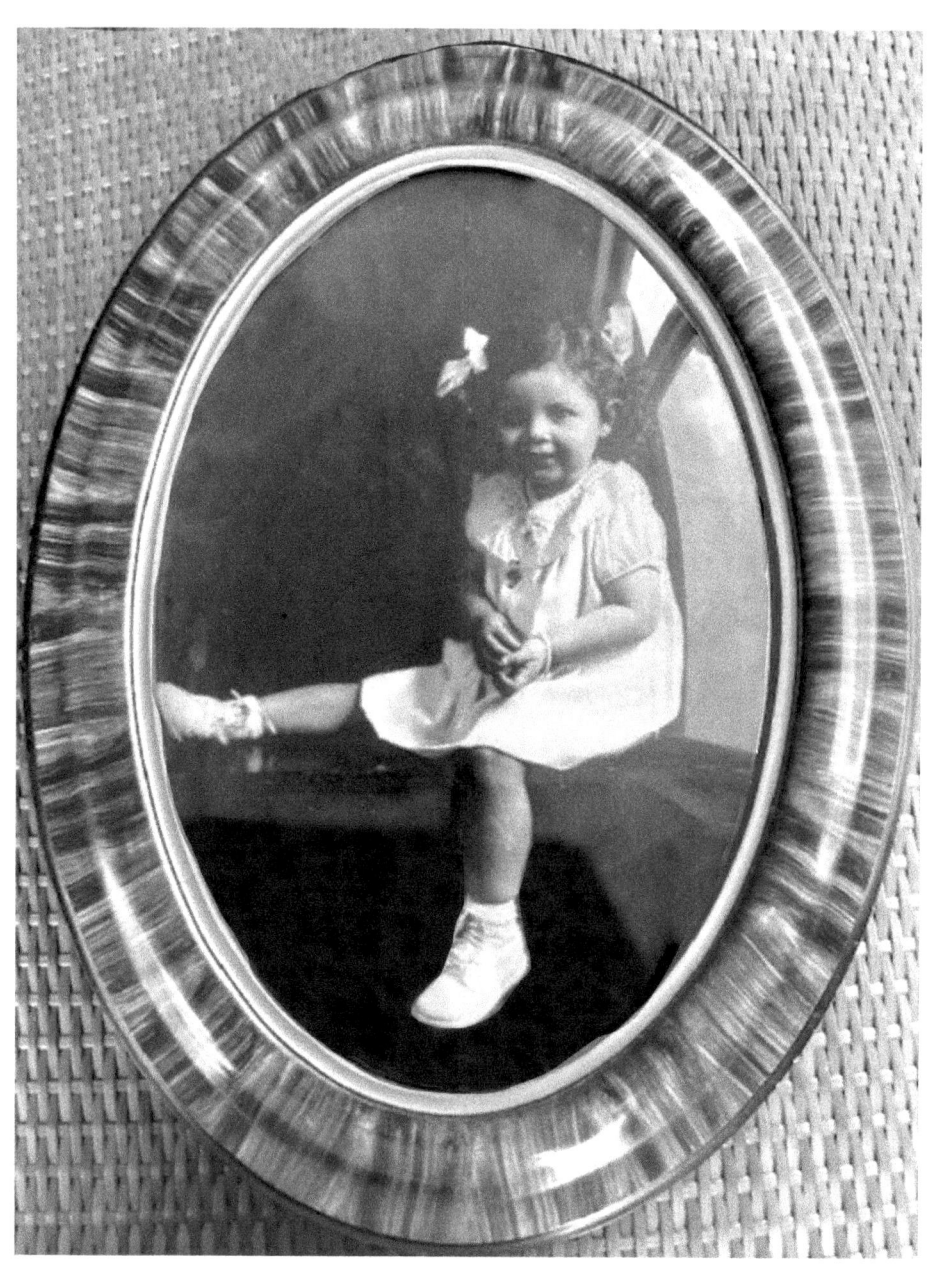

Mary as a young girl

The Story Begins

I was born, Mary W. Reis. The "W" stands for Winifred, a name that I severely disliked. I seldom let people know what the "W" stood for.

I arrived into this world on May 3, 1935, with a mixed ancestry of Portuguese and Irish/English. My father's family had come from the Portuguese island of Faial in the Azores. My mother was an Irish immigrant from Preston in the northwest part of England. We lived on the second floor of a tenement house, called a "cold water flat" in New Bedford, Massachusetts, which meant it had no hot running water. I was my parent's only surviving child, since my older brother had died at six months, supposedly from a bad case of measles.

Early in my life, my mother ended up in a serious state of depression, possibly because of her remorse over my brother's death. That did not stop us, though, from taking long walks, sometimes to one of the local parks where I enjoyed feeding the squirrels. My mother was not a great cook, so my father did a lot of the cooking. Frequently we would visit my Portuguese grandmother for meals, which I remember as being wonderful. My mother and father always loved me and spoiled me to the extent they could afford. My life as a child of a family with meager means was as serene as could be. Since I was an only child, you might even say that I was spoiled, despite our financial circumstances. That is what my husband would say.

It was interesting, that with my mother having both Irish and English relatives, we had all kinds of English memorabilia in the house including souvenirs from Queen Elizabeth's coronation.

I never went out of the house on St. Patrick's Day without "the wearing of the Green." My mother would recount her experience when she had worn the "Green" and another girl was wearing the "Orange." Even though I was very attached to my father, my Irish and English background was imbued in me. I used to tease my mother by imitating both her and her friends, but in reality, I loved to follow the Irish and some English traditions. I could have easily been a High Tea with a cucumber sandwich-type person. Green became my favorite color. My family life, unlike my husband's, was quite serene, so I will not dwell on it.

I was a very good student, and as such, was passed directly from second grade to fourth grade. My husband used to joke that I was kicked up, rather than promoted. I should never have taught him to joke. As I grew, I was a very social person with numerous neighborhood and school friends. I used to fascinate people because I could write backwards with both hands as a parlor trick. I also confused boys, especially when we played tennis with them. I would switch hands to return the ball because I had a weak backhand, and the ball, with the forehand spin, would go in a different direction than they thought. The boys I played with did not like to lose to a girl. I of course enjoyed beating them.

At New Bedford High School, I chose what was called a Commercial Curriculum. I chose this because I knew my parents could not afford to send me to a school of higher education. I became class treasurer, a member of the honor society, and a member of the senior class book committee, along with other school clubs. In today's world, I probably would have been showered with scholarships

In The Eyes of an Alzheimer's Patient

for just about any school in the country with the right curriculum. But that was yesterday, and our family needed money to survive.

I was thoroughly delighted with my time in high school and kept in contact with many of my classmates throughout my life. When the original reunion chairman was retiring from his position, thinking that the reunions were probably over because of our advanced ages, I picked it up even though we were living out of town. I felt strongly that our class should stay in touch. I continued to keep the class together for a few more years until my illness took over my life.

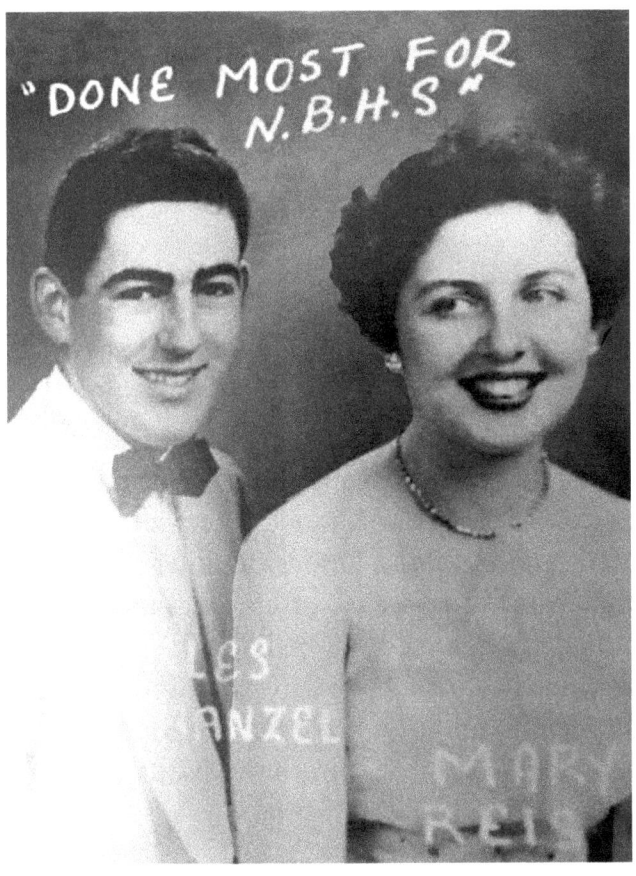

Mary Damm (Reis) selected as
"Done the most for New Bedford High School"

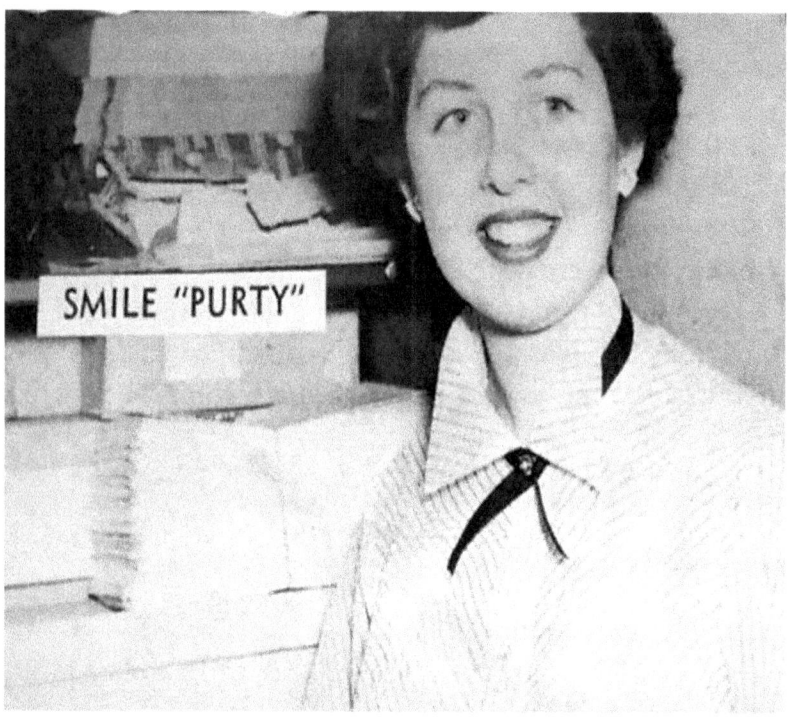

Mary is Smile "Purty"

My soon to be husband was also a good student, but very subdued. I suspect that it was because he was a relatively poor boy and had an inferiority complex. Although he was always considered a bright student and got good grades, he did so without working as conscientiously as I did because of his great memory. At this stage, he only studied hard in school if he liked the subject or the teacher. He was also mostly a visual learner. Anything that did not interest him did not seem to find its way to the memory bank. I learned what selective hearing meant at the times we discussed doing something around the house.

I happened to live close to one of Gene's two friends, so we saw each other occasionally. We also joined a youth group at the local Episcopal Church, since that is where one of his friends and one of my closest friends belonged. During this period, there was not even a hint of dating. We were just two Catholic teens in a protestant youth group, which was probably scandalous at the time.

I did not know why, but he fascinated me. Perhaps that is why he was my date for the senior prom. We were both intelligent, but he was usually outwardly calm about everything, and not very talkative to people he did not know well. I had a flash temper and was somewhat bipolar. After a severe outbreak I would confuse people, especially my husband, by acting like nothing happened. I also was not one of those "forgive, but not forget" people. I genuinely forgave and forgot many disagreements within minutes of their occurring, and would change from foe to friend, which fascinated my husband even after he got to know me later in our marriage. The anger character trait, associated with Alzheimer's, was exacerbated with my disease and would manifest itself with people I never would have normally offended. The kind people they were, usually forgave me, and blamed it, rightfully so, on my illness. My husband was usually the whipping boy for my tantrums, but he still continued his love for me. Why shouldn't he?

My husband Eugene (Gene) Philip Damm Jr. was also born in New Bedford on June 9, 1934, and lived in a "cold water flat" as well. That was the same day, month, and year as Donald Duck was "born" to the world. In later years, when his personality changed, Gene would later joke that it was the reason that he was such a quack. He disliked being called Junior and also had a dislike for the name Eugene. He is happiest when he is called Gene, which he usually uses unless it is on a legal or formal document.

His mother was a combination of Portuguese and New England Yankee, with a heritage going back to the Mayflower. His maternal grandfather was definitely on the poor side of the family that had risen as high as serving as a United States Ambassador. His grandfather never talked about this, but Gene found out about it later in life. His maternal grandfather was a staunch and feisty New England Yankee.

Gene Damm

Gene's mother was the only one in both our families who had a high school education. His paternal grandfather had arrived in this country from France where the gendarmes were looking for him. He was a glass chemist who had developed two formulas for glass that had won medals at an exposition. When his employer took credit for the gold medal, and he only received a bronze medal for his second formula, he left France with both formulas which were secret at the time. In America, he started a glass company and a fairly large family with a woman of French Canadian descent.

Unfortunately, his paternal grandfather was supposedly out drinking one night and while walking home he was killed by an automobile. The family was left with little to survive on.

Gene's father loved to tell the story of how he and one of his brothers were asked to walk their new born sister in her baby carriage. During the walk they met a boy they knew that was riding a bicycle. They did not have a bicycle, but they had another sister, so they made a trade. This trade was quickly reversed once they got home. There were many antics he talked about which met with my displeasure. To his credit, Gene's father was a very hard worker and Gene never forgot this.

Gene had a very humble childhood. His father worked for a while for the Work Projects Administration, a government program to build public facilities such libraries, parks, etc., that enabled the unemployed to earn their keep. One time, his father's check arrived on a weekend when the banks were closed. His parent's attempts to cash it at a grocery store failed. The meal that day was ketchup on bread. His mother was crying on the bed because she was the last to eat, but only if there was enough bread left from his father's, Gene's, and his two sister's meals (Claire the oldest, and Shirley the youngest of the three). At one point, Gene's bed was an old sofa in the main area of the house, near an unbearably hot coal stove blasting away to keep the rest of the house warm. His parents and two sisters occupied the other bedrooms. Gifts and clothing were at a minimum during this period.

One day, Gene did something wrong and his father chased him around the house with a ketchup bottle in his hand. When he could not catch up with him, he hit Gene in the elbow with the bottle. It hit a nerve and Gene thought that he would lose the use of his arm. Even though much as this would not be tolerated in today's world, Gene always felt that if he did wrong that he deserved to be punished. It would have been better though, if his father had caught him and spanked him with the ubiquitous strap that was kept in many of the households of that day and age. That was not overly strong punishment in those days, but it was akin to a sea captain ordering a seaman to be given 40 lashes for doing a misdeed. While not as cruel as the lashing, being hit by the bottle was still extremely painful. "Spare the rod and spoil the child" was the slogan those days. I guess that I was lucky that I was spoiled by my parents.

His father finally found a permanent job moving molten metal by hand on chains from a blast furnace. Unfortunately, his parent's marriage did not last and they ended up in divorce. This was more unusual than it is today and Gene was embarrassed to tell people, especially when an instructor questioned him strongly in front of his high school class for not having both parents sign a form. The teacher was sorry he had asked the question after hearing Gene's tearful answer in front of the whole class. The damage, though, was done. For Gene, it was a lesson in life that you should learn not to put things in a way that you inadvertently and wrongly upset people, especially when you do not have all the facts. He could not go on class trips because of the expense. Gene was more of a follower than a leader at that time in his life. I helped with much of his personality change. In later life, Gene was able to drift back and forth on personalities, depending on the situation, even sometimes to his detriment. If he was in the right situation, he could joke about things, but that was so rare that it went unnoticed by most people who knew him then. Now it is more common, and he teases and jokes a lot. I think that I created a monster.

He had a severe astigmatism and wore glasses at an early age. He also had very little coordination and athletic skills. He did play basketball for the Protestant church league team, with the group we belonged to, but was not very good at it. He also did not know anything about skills around the house as he always lived in rentals. Except for his eyesight, his coordination and handyman skills improved in time.

Gene's maternal grandfather lived with them at one point, staying in the same bedroom as Gene. He helped with many expenses such as buy clothes for Gene and his two sisters . He also took Gene to Red Sox ballgames. Bleacher tickets were cheap and you could purchase them at the game. The bus to Boston was also reasonably priced. He had a great time with his grandfather. That ended when his grandfather passed away. Gene always thought that he was spoiled more than the girls by both his mother and grandfather because he was the only boy. Gene felt that his nerdy intelligence gave them high hopes for him.

In our senior yearbook, one of the students on the committee put in the printed version of our yearbook that Gene's future fate would be in the "school of hard knocks" even though his ambition was to attend Northeastern University despite the fact that they couldn't afford it. They listed his musical trademark as "Oh, The Pity Of It All." The other graduates got more glowing reviews. Somehow these comments got by the faculty advisor for the yearbook. This is a reminder to anyone that may still be poring over it or reading this book of how people could joke at that period in time and how openly cruel and wrong they could be.

I, who was one of the most popular and interactive girls in our class, ended up marrying the boy who seemed most likely not to succeed. His review may have seemed true to them, but it was cruel to him.

With all my activities, I was selected as the female who did most for the school, for our class yearbook. In Gene's eyes, they had me pegged right as a freelance writer, but I never pursued that, much to Gene's regret. I did write a children's story one time, which people who saw it loved it, but I never submitted it for publication regardless of Gene's encouragement.

Look at the vivid contrast between my active high school life and Gene's to understand the difference in the social life we lived at the time.

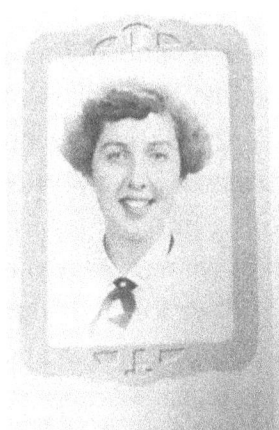

MARY WINIFRED REIS
Alias: "*Winnie*"   May 3
367 Earle St.
Activities and Honors: Class Treasurer 2, 3, 4; Assistant Editor Crimson Log 4; Honor Society 3, 4; Allied Youth 3; Square Dance Club 3; Dramatic Club 3; Crimson Courier Reporter 3; Junior Red Cross 3; Secretary Guidance Office 4; Steering Committee 3, 4.
Future Ambition: Free Lance Writer
Probable Fate: Multi-Millionaire at Seventeen (Class Dues where did you go?)
Musical Trademark: "Brother Can You Spare A Dime."

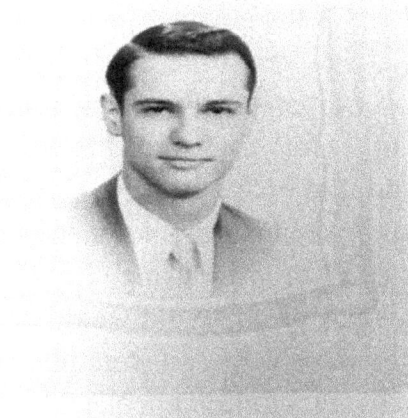

EUGENE PHILIP DAMM
Alias: "*Gene*"   June 9
203 Tinkham St.
Activities and Honors: Math Club 2.
Future Ambition: Northeastern
Probable Fate: School of Hard Knocks
Musical Trademark: "Oh, The Pity Of It All"

Gene Damm

The beginning of Our Adventures Together

The boy that I dated in my senior year was quiet and shy, and very different from my extrovert personality. Regardless of our differences, we eventually fell in true love. We had known each other for years since I lived close to one of his friends. We all hung around each other like a gang. In the summer, going into our senior year in high school, we started dating. I think that we were starting to fall in love during our senior year, but little did we know at our senior prom, that it would be a date that would last for many years. In some ways, we were like Jack Spratt and his wife in the nursery rhyme. I loved chocolate, he did not. I liked fatty foods, and he did not. I loved olives, and he hated them. I organized my work on paper, and he used his brain to keep track of things and hated paperwork. I had lots of friends, and he only had two. I don't know why we meshed so well, but we did. Maybe we did because he never took my chocolate and olives. He did succumb to going to events with my friends since the rest of his social life after school was minimal.

Both of us had small incomes from part-time jobs. Gene worked every day after school, as well as all day Saturday at a shoe store until 9:00 PM. He was paid 50 cents an hour which was below minimum wage even for mercantile work, but it was a job.

In The Eyes of an Alzheimer's Patient

I had a job at a dress shop as its bookkeeper during my high school years. The hours were better than Genes and I also ran the store if the owners were not able to be there. We had limited time together but enjoyed every minute of it. Some of our friends had cars, so we did get to go some places together. One of my friend's boyfriends used to pick her up alone with me and Gene and we would go somewhere after we finished our rehearsal of the Messiah for the city choir. We sang the Messiah annually on Christmas Eve and thoroughly enjoyed it.

During my senior year in high school, my father lost his job driving a truck for a wholesale grocery company when it went out of business. He was given very little compensation for his years of service, and for the rest of his life, he worked part-time jobs in order to support our family. After graduation, I got a job at a coal company as a bookkeeper working on a manual bookkeeping machine. Talk about muscles. I quickly became the head bookkeeper and was able to help my parents with the everyday expenses.

After Gene's parent's divorce, his mother eventually remarried and moved away. Gene did not move with his mother because he was attending school. His two sisters did leave with her though. Gene lived with his father and his father's new wife for a short while, but the apartment was not suitable for a young man who was up late. It was a "rabbit run apartment," over a fish market, where he had to pass through his father and stepmother's bedroom to get to his room, even late at night. He eventually ended up living with his great aunt and uncle.

His great aunt Bertha, was an incredible force in his life as she treated him like a son. She made homemade soups, to his delight, and fed him well. When she did not have time to make him lunch, she gave him money which he used to buy lunch at a diner near the school. She insisted that her children take her to our daughter's weddings, from New Bedford Massachusetts to Fishkill, New York at age 92, even though it was a long trip for her. As frail as she was at the time of the wedding, she had told her family that if they were not going to take her there, she would take a bus. That settled that. Her family loved her, and they were not going to allow her to make the trip alone. The bond between her and my husband was very strong and they knew it. She was like a mother to him, and he was like a son to her. In later years, Gene was not one to miss swimming meets, especially championship meets, but when she passed away, he had his Athletic Director at Vassar College watch over the teams for Friday night at a championship meet. He drove to Massachusetts and returned on Saturday after the funeral. That is how strong the bond was between them. An interesting fact was when her sister had died, she had promised her mother that she would marry her sister's husband to bring up his children. What an unselfish woman.

Gene could not afford commutation as well as tuition at most colleges, but he so much wanted to continue his education. He looked at the Naval ROTC, but at the time, they would not take people with glasses into the program, and he had that severe astigmatism. He could not have been able to handle the associated costs including travel anyway.

His two friends were looking at a small college in New Bedford and Gene went with them to see what it was like. The tuition was cheap, about $100 per semester, and it was a commuter school. Gene had a path to a college education and took it. He had a limited selection of fields, none of which were in fields he would have chosen as his career if he'd had an option. But there was no option. I liked it because he could continue dating me from a local school. We dated through his college career. Gene was taking a technical writing course and the professor would point out to the class how well his papers captured the technical analysis of a subject, but all the same, he was not getting A's. I decided that I should type his papers since his handwriting was so bad. After that, he received the grade of A for his papers. He apparently had lost points for what the instructor thought was sloppy handwriting and did not tell Gene the reason for the deduction. I won't comment on that. The professor was an excellent instructor and Gene appreciated that.

Gene was recruited to join the college's Honor Society, but he turned it down because of the requirements to do some community service. He felt that with his work schedule and spending so much time with me, he could not fulfill the additional responsibility. I wonder how many people would be that conscientious.

In Gene's senior year of college, we decided that we would get married while he was still in school. I of course decided that it was a good idea, made the suggestion, and set the date. The alternative was to wait until he graduated, but then he might have a job that took him away from home, and me. How would he have survived without me? Decent jobs in our hometown were not available at the time, and accepting a job out of town might delay our wedding plans. A school year was a better choice. April 19, 1956 was chosen since it was a holiday in Massachusetts and we both had the day off and the attendees were all available.

Guess who planned all that. Later in life, my oldest son-in-law heard me say the word "we" in a conversation, even though I was the one who was responsible. He asked if that was the "royal we." Of course, he was right. That term was used in future conversations, and I loved it. I ruled the house, and Gene always agreed to things I committed him to, even without waiting for him to step up or asking him first.

The wedding was a quiet one at Saint Kilian's church, and we had a small reception at the local Portuguese club. My husband's great aunt, whom he was still living with at the time, had baked two turkeys in her oil-fed, double oven cookstove, which she made into sandwiches for the wedding party. My aged grandmother had hit the numbers, which were popular at the time, albeit illegal, and donated the money she made to defray expenses, so we were able to buy some sandwiches, bottled beer, and soda for the guests. That, along with a jukebox playing recordings, comprised the reception banquet.

Gene Damm

    We had enough money saved up for a weekend in New York City at a commuter hotel. My girlfriend's father took us to the train station. That was our grand honeymoon. Afterwards it was right back to work and school. Gene's classmates had attended the wedding reception and asked the professor to reschedule a test he was going to give them until Gene got back from our honeymoon. The professor asked Gene when he arrived back whether he wanted to extend that. Gene said no, even though he had not studied on our honeymoon. Guess who got the best grade? Gene does not like to be vainglorious, but he relished that grade.

In The Eyes of an Alzheimer's Patient

Gene Damm

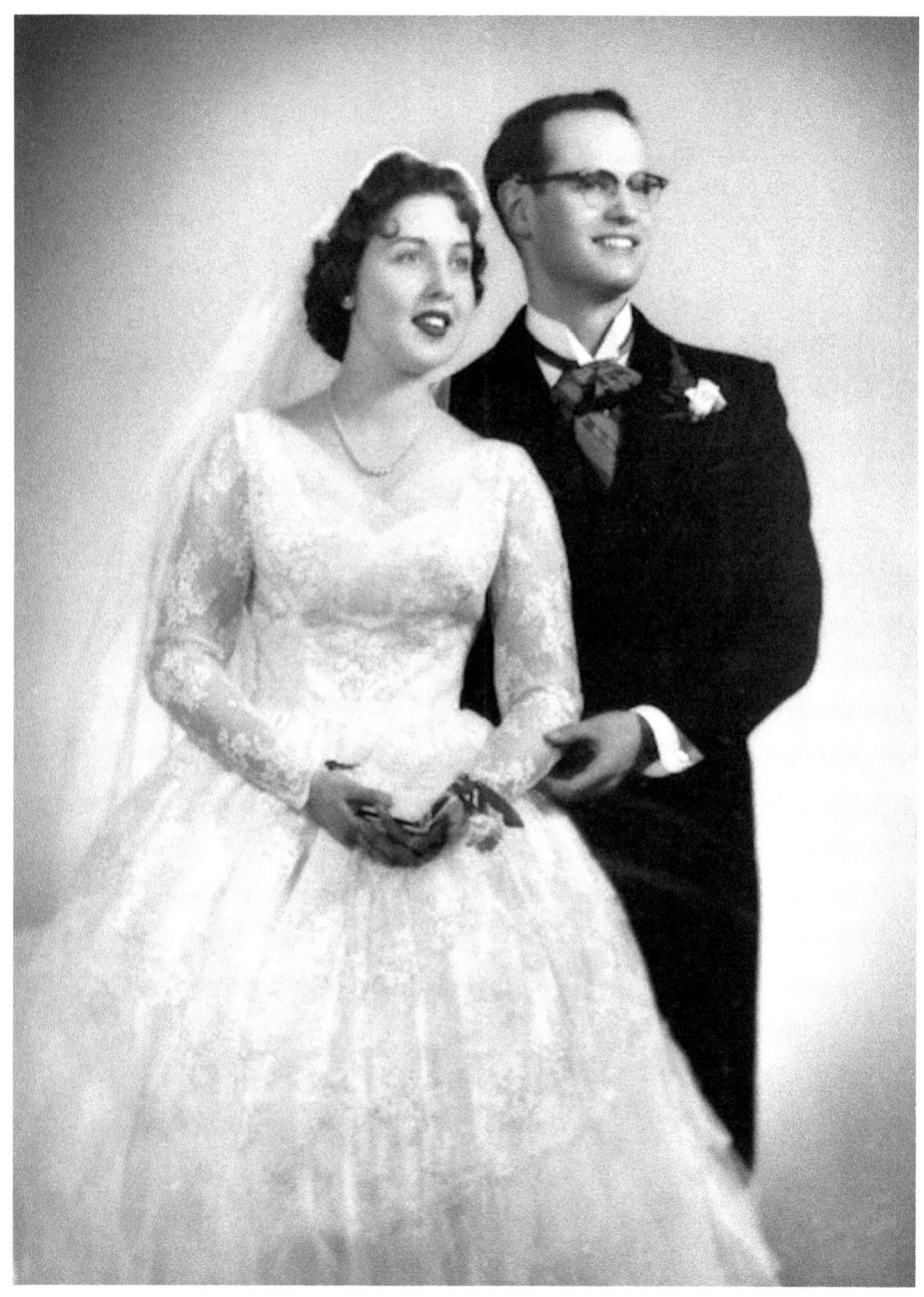

Our Early Life Together

My husband graduated quite high at the undergraduate level and was given an award from the American Textile and Colorists Association as one of the outstanding graduates in that field. His name, along with those of graduates of other schools, appeared in their national yearbook. I was so proud of him. He was also offered a Teaching Fellowship, with free tuition and a stipend, from Dartmouth College, an Ivy League school, to get his master's degree in organic chemistry. This was unusual, to say the least, coming from a school without accreditation in traditional chemistry, especially when his degree was in Textile Chemistry which was the only chemistry degree the college offered. Most of the other curricula, except mechanical engineering, were in the textile field and did not carry with them a bachelor's degree,

Things were falling in place even though he really did not want to be a chemist. Gene would have preferred to be a lawyer or a newspaper reporter. He never really told this to anybody, except around the time when he was working on this book. Do you think that I had a role in his revealing this part of the story? I will never tell.

Gene had already been considered for a full-time job at a major chemical company, and when he told them he was going to graduate school, they immediately offered him a summer job. He turned it down so we could spend the summer at home. I would keep my job at the coal company, and he would keep his job at the shoe store.

During the summer I was expecting our first child, the unexpected happened. The shoe store said that they did not need him for that summer. What a shock this was for both of us. He had worked there through his high school and college years. Now that he had the responsibility of a family, they released him. Fortunately, one of his friend's fathers knew the mayor and he and his two friends went to city hall and got jobs in the cemetery department where they would be trimming gravesites. Eventually, a lawn mowing job opened up, and Gene took it because it paid more than trimming the graves. When the allotted weeks were used up, the shoe store decided that they needed Gene after all, and gave him back his old job. All that, plus my pay at the coal company helped pay for our summer apartment and food, with a little left over.

I had readily agreed, before this all happened, that moving to Hanover, New Hampshire to attend Dartmouth College was the right thing to do. It was a great honor. There was also no question about us doing this to fulfill Gene's dream of advanced education. We were in this together, like we would live the rest of our life, as a team. I wanted him to fulfill his dream, as much as he did, even though it meant hard work and sacrifices. We needed to be very frugal with our spending, but with the confidence of youth, we felt that we could make things work. The father of one of his friends drove us and a little furniture to the college. We lived in reconverted Naval ROTC duplex homes on sticks rather than foundations. The weather was rather cold, in a climate where the temperature reached 26 below zero one winter. During the winter months, we banked snow against the side of the house to keep us warmer and use less fuel. Our heater was an oil stove without burner wicks, so you would trickle in the oil and stand back as the stove rumbled if the pool of oil was too large. The heat did not stop the shower drain and shower from filling up with water until the warmth of the warm water melted the ice beneath it. Life was tough, but we were not accustomed to frivolities anyway and survived for those two years.

We had our first-born child, Mary Catherine, there while we were still on thin rations. Fortunately, my former employer carried my health insurance, without any cost, until we had the baby. It was still tough financially, with a newborn, but we survived. I had taken part-time jobs at the college typing recaps of presentations and typing master's and PhD theses on a very old manual typewriter. Most of these jobs were a result of an interview at the college employment office when we first arrived on campus. They were very good at finding work for wives of graduate students. During the interview, I had mentioned that I was expecting a child in the event that it would impact some of the jobs that they might offer. The interviewer expressed his amazement at my being so honest and said that he was not used to the wives telling him about their situation until they had to leave the job. He kept giving me typing jobs as he found them.

My first job was typing the minutes of a lecture series on the students and the college. Dartmouth College was an all-male school at the time and since there was no recording of the lectures, I needed to attend all the lectures. It was just me and all those male freshmen. The shorthand that I was taught in high school really came in handy. After that, the jobs were sporadic since I was typing from home, but even the little money I received helped us greatly. One of the assignments was to type the Ph.D. thesis for one of the professors. When I finished a section, he would travel to Harvard to get it reviewed. It was in sociology, so I could understand most of it and it was a natural for me. The only problem was that he would present each section before he initially planned to go to get that section reviewed. Then he would not come back for it for a week or two. So much for rushing it. One day he saw our daughter in her playpen and asked what her name was. I said, Mary Catherine. He said that he had a son and I asked him his son's name and he said "Adam, the first boy." Wouldn't you know that chosen name would come from the logic of a sociologist? I wonder what his wife was thinking.

Gene Damm

With no car at the time, we shopped at either the local cooperative grocery store, called "The Coop for food," or the small grocery store alternative in town. Food and good shoes for the baby, when she was old enough to wear them, were our major expenses on a tough budget. The town was very small. I and another graduate student's wife walked its' length many times with our babies. Our only transportation that year was by bus. Once, on a trip home from Hanover, we had a stop in Boston near a restaurant to wait for the next bus. Mary Catherine was hungry, and I convinced Gene to see if they could warm up her milk bottle. The word we got was that we made the chef's day. They were nice people at a restaurant where we were obviously not going to eat. The next year we got our licenses and bought a used car for $75 from someone who had lost their license. That became our new mode of transportation.

We were used to going with the flow. We had to make do with whatever the circumstances presented. We were the generation that was told if we dropped some candy on the ground, we were told to pick it up, because we were going to eat a pound of dirt before we died anyway. Buying new candy was not an option. We were also the generation of lead paint on the walls. In one place my husband had lived as a child, a pipe in the kitchen needed replacing. They found that the old pipe was a lead one, which still smelled of the gas that it had carried at one time. I wonder now what might have been different for us if we did not come into contact with what now would be considered somewhat deadly, and mind-destroying. We were tough and resilient. We were also the generation where some children wore bags of camphor around their neck to ward off disease. I am not sure how well it did this, but with the strong camphor smell it may have been the first successful practice of social distancing.

Prior to graduation, my husband was offered a great job with IBM with an equally great salary, which was higher than other graduate students, even one who had two years prior industrial experience. It was probably the most respected company in the world at the time and Gene loved working for them. He was a loyal employee throughout his career. Curiously enough, they were interested in his background in textile chemistry for a product they were developing. The climb up the wall of happiness had begun. It was still tough in the beginning, because, we had one, then two, then three children to care for, and little family financial support to build up a household on a single salary. But we did it, even eventually paying for three college educations, without any debt on our children's part. Most of the time, I was a stay-at-home mother who managed our money (and Gene). Gene used to quip that if he ever would have to sign his own checks that he would be arrested for forgery. Our daughters were Mary, Erin, and Kathleen. Mary's name was supposed to add Catherine to Mary, in my mind, but we had not joined the two, and she is forever just Mary.

I had a fetish for dressing the girls exactly alike. They looked like different sized triplets. Later, someone also noticed that in our casual dress, Gene and I had the same jackets at times. I wonder why? I also would not let my children out of the house on Saint Patrick's Day without having something green on them. My Irish heritage was a very important side of me. I also liked beer, whether in a glass or a bottle. It was my favorite drink at an Irish Pub while eating my fish and chips. Gene did not like bottled beer at the time, and still would prefer draft beer, if he were to drink at all. Yet another one of our differences.

He did not drink in college, even on the occasions where his fellow students drank ample glasses of it from a keg that they had bought. They convinced Gene to go with them to buy the keg, even though he was the non-drinker, because he had a heavy beard even when he shaved.

One holiday, when my father offered him an alcoholic drink and he turned it down, my father tried to encourage him by saying that, "You might as well be drunk, as the way you are now." Oh well, that was my Gene, and that was my father.

Gene Damm

Our Family Life and Gene's Career

Endicott, New York was the first stop in our lifelong adventures. Gene was doing very well in his job. He had a wonderful first appraisal and was promoted in six months to the next level. The only flaw noted was that he was too quiet, a trait he was more than able to overcome, thanks partly to me.

He also had his first patent there. It was in the field of attracting liquids through the air in the shape of a character formed by an electric field imposed on them. This fascinated him and he became quite knowledgeable in what electric fields can do, as you will see later.

During that time in Endicott, we had a couple of our so called, bumps in the road. Gene was on a business trip in Ohio, when the house we were renting at the time was flooded in a massive rain storm. Employees from the utility company rescued my father and mother who were staying with us, as well as myself and our two young daughters. They had to break through the screen door, since the water was close to waist high at that point. We were also expecting our third daughter within the next two months, so it was a traumatic experience. The rescuers moved us to a neighbor's house at higher ground. Gene was not immediately informed about the incident, but the coworker with him on the trip was notified. Without telling Gene about the incident until they arrived back at Endicott, he was able to reschedule their flight to an earlier one.

We were safe and Gene moved us into a local hotel for the night. However, when the water from the storm receded, the house and furnishings were covered in mud. His fellow employees, including his second-level manager's wife, helped us salvage as much as we could. We stayed in a trailer that a friend of his owned for a few months until we found another place to rent. Meanwhile, Gene was stricken with a number of staph infections from the flood, as a result of his weakened resistance from the cleanup effort. It took a while to get over these "adverse events."

Prior to the flood, I was so depressed with the challenges of our family that I became a hypochondriac. Our doctor was very dedicated and came to our house frequently to take care of me. During one visit, I asked him why he charged us so little. He laughed and said that he would make it up on the next IBM'er that could better afford it. For some reason, the flood seemed to jar me back to my senses of responsibility and all was well again.

We eventually were able buy a small house in the Endwell area, a suburb of Endicott. We had one share of IBM stock, bought with a discount on the employee stock plan, and used that as a down payment.

Another bump in the road occurred when I developed scarlet fever, pneumonia, and a large lung abscess about the size of a small orange. The surgeon wanted to operate on it to close the gap that it produced. I did not want that, and my family doctor supported my position, at least temporarily. I had them bring my statues of Saints to the hospital, and of course there were lots of prayers. One day our doctor walked into the hospital looking like he needed a shave and said that he had just returned from a Russian monastery in Pennsylvania where he had said a prayer for all his patients. He was known to reschedule his late visits to someone's house to the morning rather than waking up the children.

Church members and friends watched the children, and provided food and essentials, so Gene could take that time to visit me. They also mowed the lawn for him. Suddenly the abscess scarred over and there were no visible signs of it slowing down my activity. Again, we were on the road to happiness.

There was a little humor in our life with an incident at the Catholic Church we attended. Our two youngest daughters always fought over who would sit in the seat next to the aisle. One day Gene told them that neither one was going to sit there, so they would go in first. They obediently did that, but since we were early and the rest of the pew was empty, they proceeded to go to the other side. Knowing that they were probably in trouble, they moved all the way to the end of the pew and sat on the baseboard heating unit. We internally laughed knowing that we shouldn't. Then came the "Oh no moment." It was a Holy Day when the priest walked down the side aisle right by the girls. The Church was filled at that point, so it was not totally embarrassing, and we eventually laughed about it.

Gene eventually was offered a job in Poughkeepsie, New York which was closer to my parent's apartment in Massachusetts. We, and I emphasize we, accepted it. It was there, upon the promotion of his manager, that Gene started his management career. When the project moved to Boulder, Colorado, Gene did not want to move, especially since I would not have liked that. He did agree for both of us to visit Boulder, while he consulted about the transfer of his earlier work. After the visit, we remained adamant that we were not going to move. I was the dominant factor again, but you will see how this changed dramatically when we coached together.

Gene became manager of the Chemistry lab in Poughkeepsie. He built the lab up with all kinds of equipment such as x-ray, an electron microscope, and a nuclear magnetic resonance unit. In those day, it was very sophisticated equipment and rare for a small laboratory to have them. He also had an advance technology group there, and he started up a study in using electric fields to attract small particles in fluids, that could coat electronic parts flawlessly, when other methods failed. It was similar to something used in the automotive industry, and Gene thought that they could develop something for electronics. This became his new way in using electricity to move things to where they could be useful. The process was called electrophoretic deposition for lack of a better name. Don't ask me what that means. It was affectionately called, the EPD process by a PhD chemical engineer who worked for Gene in honor of the work that Gene had done in this area. They were Gene's initials. He reminded Gene of this for years after he left IBM.

At the time Gene and his advanced technology group were working on the EPD project, IBM had trouble with the corrosion of contacts on the core memory stacks in their computers. They were having considerable corrosion on the stack connectors when their computers were used in the paper and oil industries. Millions were at stake. Coating them by other means was not perfect. They then turned to the process that Gene had directed his group to develop as a means of solving the problem. Since the contacts were metal, and required only ten volts to coat them, it was a perfect way to cover the smallest part without leaving holes. Gene was awarded an Outstanding Contribution Award which was later upgraded to a Corporate Award.

The girls were getting older and I loved it. Having three girls was the thrill my life as they got older. I now had real life dolls that I would lavish with pretty dresses. Gene accepted my follies in buying clothes, but he commented on the fact that the wife of our next-door neighbor, who was reasonably well off, asked to borrow one of our oldest daughter's gowns. I also had a fetish that they should not do anything that was considered "mans" work. Gene was not getting any help with work projects from my daughters. They were to be brought up as real ladies. I also wanted them to have the college education that I was lacking at the time with no expense to them.

Gene Damm

During his career at IBM, Gene received a number of awards, such as five Invention Achievement awards, the Corporate Outstanding Contribution award, where we were both treated to a stay at the famous Plaza Hotel in New York City along with tickets to a Broadway show of our choice, and a Good Management award. At the Corporate Award get-together we were told that before the show of our choice, we could go to any restaurant we wanted to and eat whatever was on the menu. His manager's recommendation was Chateaubriand. Being simple people, we had a rush dinner at Mama Leone's before the show. The Invention Achievement Awards came as a result of accumulating points for patents, and other inventions, which were placed in a special publication to prevent other companies from patenting them. At one point early in his technical career, when IBM had its own national magazine, Gene was mentioned as one of the up-and-coming inventors at IBM.

All awards came with money, and large framed certificates, so the wall of happiness was building higher.

He advanced quickly to a senior level rank, which was the highest technical rank one could receive at a laboratory, in an unusual way. When his manager achieved that rank, one of Gene's fellow workers told Gene that he had deserved it rather than his manager. Gene did not worry about that, because he felt that his manager would take care of him, at least financially, and told him that. His fellow employee probably thought he was crazy. However, in a few months, Gene was promoted to the same level as his manager. It was unusual, but his faith in his manager was justified. At one point the laboratory director wanted Gene to go to a fancy California resort for a week with him to work on a particular project which was of no interest to Gene. He did not want to travel, so he sent one of the managers who reported to him. The laboratory director was not happy about that since he had wanted to treat Gene with a vacation. But as you will see later, all was forgiven. Gene did not want to travel and was happy to be home with me and the girls. The girls and I were more important to him.

In The Eyes of an Alzheimer's Patient

As a manager, he always felt, in tough meetings, that he wanted to meet with others in his office. He felt that being behind his desk gave him a psychological advantage. It didn't hurt that they had to look at all his large framed award certificates mounted on the wall behind him. Typical Gene, when he had achieved a management level that he could have a rug in his office, he had his secretary decide on the color. Making technical and management decisions were much easier than deciding the color of his rug. I would have made a great secretary for him. I could type, protect him from unwanted visitors, and openly tell him tell him exactly what was his best approach to a management problem.

His friends also meant more to him than their title. A couple of his secretaries even visited our house and talked to us like we were old friends. One even did this after Gene moved from that job.

We did not choose our friends based on race, color, creed, or status. One of my close friends was the wife of a man that Gene went to graduate school with. We had even bought our new house near them. He ended up working for Gene, in his advance technology group. When we invited them to our Christmas party, the wife called me and asked if we should do this because of the circumstances. We said essentially that they were our friends, knowing that Gene could separate our personal relationship with them from his work relationship. We had a number of other friends, including a friend from our Church, that Gene really liked. He had a large family, and we enjoyed vacationing with them. To this day, Gene remembers him as one of his best friends.

While Gene was busy at work, I was busy bringing up our daughters, as well as taking care of my parents. My parent's care was initially remote and through frequent visits by both of us to help them take care of themselves. I was very active in our daughter's school parent's organization, and eventually Gene got involved by setting up guest speakers and starting up a science fair, as well as a speaker's bureau for the school.

Gene Damm

Gene was eventually promoted to division headquarters where he was responsible for funding technology projects at most of the IBM laboratories across the United States and Europe. One of the projects came as a result of being asked by the division president to look at the use of fiber optics in military aircrafts, by IBM's Federal Systems Division. He saw the potential and helped fund the first study in the use of fiber optics in IBM's product development arm.

He took risks at IBM, of which I never thought he was capable. As the Advanced Technology Manager, a title at division headquarters, which carried more prestige than authority, he sent a memo telling laboratories in the United States and Europe to get rid of PCBs in their capacitors. PCBs were suspected carcinogens in Japan and were brought to his attention by a friend working in IBM's World Trade organization.

Prior to sending the memo out to replace the old capacitors with new ones, he funded a laboratory site to develop a substitute. When the director for one of the major manufacturing divisions refused to comply with the laboratories request to change the capacitors, Gene was told about it. He said that he would write a letter to that manufacturing division president. Shortly after that, he received a call from the director, upset that he heard Gene was going to write such a letter. Gene's response was something like, "Certainly. I am in the process of writing it now. I will read it to you." The director was devastated about the effects of PCBs and convinced of the importance of replacing the capacitors when he heard the reasoning behind the decision. It saved an argument of polarized views, and Gene favored that way.

Unlike the liquid PCBs in the old capacitors, the liquid in the new capacitor, while environmentally safer, was flammable, so a special fuse was added to the system that would break the circuit if it got too warm. Gene had used his nice sounding title to successfully get the sites in the United States and Europe that his division controlled, to use the new and more environmentally suitable capacitor. This worked out well, even though Gene stepped out his role of technology into the world of product development. He could have lost his job by not turning his study and solution for a new capacitor over to product development management. Maybe he should have consulted with me on that one.

At one point Gene thought he might actually be fired if the division president was informed that they had to store the PCB capacitors in warehouses until they found a way to dispose of the non-flammable liquid. Then the headlines hit about a company dumping the potentially toxic chemical in the Hudson River. Had he notified the division president of what he was doing, he would have been a hero. But that's not Gene. Unlike some people who wanted to be in the eye of the president by bringing attention to their work, Gene felt that what he was doing was all included in his job responsibilities and he did not need to inform anybody, even though with such a large decision, he should have. That is my naive husband.

Among other things, I picked out his clothes, because he was not a shopper. He also did not know how to pick out complementary colors to wear. The family council still critiques him for that. Since I did it all for him, he never learned to do it himself. When he was advanced technology manager at division headquarters, he wore colorful shirts such as a vertical striped red and blue shirt and an orange shirt. His most subtle shirt was a light blue button down. I had bought him these so he wore them, even in staid IBM, the home of white shirts and wing tipped shoes. He thinks he got away with that because people thought that he was one of those intelligent crazy people who broke formality and did not care. The title helped create that image.

Eventually, because of a customer complaint on the dress code of some of IBM's service men, the message came down that white shirts were the rule. Light blue shirts were allowed because they showed up better on TV. One day when Gene saw one of his friends wearing a light blue shirt, he asked why he was wearing a colored shirt. The remark came back, "How come you are wearing a white shirt?" Guess who shopped for his white shirts? After all, I had bought the colored ones.

He did all that while commuting sixty miles each way to White Plains. I had taken a stand that we should not make a house move, even if it was paid for, while one of our daughters was of high school age and the other two were soon to follow.

During a trip to France for an extended meeting at IBM's La Gaude laboratory in the Alps, located outside of Nice, Gene was shocked to see that the Riviera beach was comprised of rocks and not sand. Gene did not like the narrow road with no guard rails going to the top of that mountain, so he always took a ride offered to him.

During another time when we traded one of our timeshares to meet with our daughter Erin and her husband Jim, we had to drive up and down a mountainside after leaving the Reno airport for a visit to Lake Tahoe. The steep road was bad enough, but coming down, negotiating the road with no guard rail and three hairpin turns, was extremely slow and harrowing. I sat in the back seat, not looking to the side, and Gene white-knuckled it back to the Reno airport. Lake Tahoe was beautiful, but the drive up and down from the Reno side was something we would not repeat.

When Gene left IBM headquarters to go back to the laboratory, which he dearly wanted to do, his old boss actually had Gene interview his potential replacements. One individual kept asking Gene how much he met with the division president. Gene essentially said that he did not meet with him because he was able to solve problems himself. The candidate pursued the subject, and it was obvious that he wanted the visibility more than the job. After the interview, Gene called his manager and told him not to hire that person.

Gene then moved to work for the laboratory director in Poughkeepsie. Even though it would seem to be a lesser job than his headquarters job, it made Gene happy to not have any more long commutes.

The laboratory director appreciated Gene's efforts so much that he insisted he be part of the senior management group to go to Puerto Rico for rest and relaxation. Gene was a workaholic and was not too happy about it, but he went and would not refuse the director again. When the director observed that Gene was still trying to work while in Puerto Rico, he told Gene to take a walk with him on the beach. He informed Gene that continuing to work from there was not in the plan. He wanted to reward him, not give him a change in his work location.

At this time, our oldest was driving, so a little of my responsibility to transport them places was eased. Wouldn't you know it, one day when the girls drove Gene to work so that they could use his car, Gene needed to work late with the laboratory director. The work ended abruptly when the guard at the front desk called the laboratory director to say that our daughters had been waiting for him in the front lobby for some time.

When the laboratory director left his job, he moaned to Gene that he regretted that he did not do more for him. Gene was very happy with the comment and repeated it to me when he got home. My comment was, "But he didn't do more for you." It was one of the few times that I spoke up on work issues.

There were other memorable events such as when Boston College was thinking of setting up an engineering program and Gene was chosen to provide the technical guidance. Gene knew a fair amount of the expenses involved in setting up an engineering program and a presentation was created contrasting computer science costs due to the emerging interest in computers and programming among high school students in the main regions from which the college drew. It was Gene's presentation which convinced Boston College to set up a master's degree program in computer science and programming rather than incurring the much greater expense of an engineering programming. Both the school and the sales staff that arranged the presentation were very pleased with the results. Helping a college from our home state produced great satisfaction.

Gene was in California at a month-long class for high potential executives, run by UCLA professors, that focused on statistics and probability as well as other sciences. At the class, he received a call from the manager who had initially brought him to division headquarters. He was offered a job with a promotion, back in Endicott. It was in a product area with which Gene was not familiar and Gene knew that I did not want to go back there, which was the main reason that he turned down the opportunity. Then the phone calls came every morning at breakfast for the rest of the month he attended the class. The waiter would come to the breakfast table each morning to announce the call. Gene made the mistake of telling the manager that if he were going to move, he would prefer a job managing the laboratory's technology efforts. It was more in his field. The next day, the laboratory director called to say that if the technology job became available, Gene would be considered for it. The condition was that he take the Endicott job that his former manager offered him first. He still turned it down even though he would have loved the technology job, mainly because I would not move back, and that was fine with Gene. However, this could have been a career-breaker.

When he arrived back at headquarters from California, his boss suggested that he visit Endicott and make peace with the offering manager, who still wanted to hire him. He even called the director of technology at division headquarters, feeling that it might save Gene's career. Rejecting jobs from strong-willed high-level managers in IBM did not bode well for one's career. Gene thought that the visit was a good idea and off he flew to Endicott for a day. His goal was to go over his position face to face with the manager who would not give up on hiring him.

In The Eyes of an Alzheimer's Patient

At the laboratory, the offering manager chose to reiterate his offer to Gene while on the way to lunch and passing a corporate vice president visiting at the site who knew Gene. The manager asked the vice president to help convince Gene to take the job. When they returned from lunch, Gene told the manager that his wife had agreed that if he took the job, he could commute to our home on weekends. Gene then told him that, while he liked the offering manager, he was not going to do that. The manager, though tough, was a good family man and respected him for it. As usual, Gene's honesty got him off the hook. Good for me that I was able to take a stand on this without hurting Gene.

He was later offered a job in Kingston reporting directly to the site manager to straighten out the education department. It was the same manager who wanted him in Endicott. It would be even more unusual to turn down a job from that manager a second time and would certainly hurt a good relationship. It was also a shorter commuting distance from our home. He took the job.

Gene at one point hosted a dinner for graduates in a master's program given at IBM Kingston through Syracuse University. The speaker was a famous science fiction writer and he was seated at our table, as Gene's department was hosting the event. This writer even wrote a poem about me and gave it to me. He may have been considered a well-known author, but he seemed somewhat too boastful to suit my taste and I never kept the poem. I choose my own friends. Thankfully, I held my tongue for Gene sake.

Gene had successfully revived the education department in Kingston and it was getting some esteem among other IBM sites and division management. The site manager was good to Gene, but he was an emotional person. Gene was told that at another IBM site he had broken many a telephone, while he was site manager there, by banging the telephone down after a conversation that did not go well. Needless to say, they had to replace several of his phones. He was still a great person in many respects. He once talked IBM out of expanding the Kingston site because a study he had created showed that if things went sour with the economy, or the business, downsizing would have too much of an impact on the area. He was not a power grabber, and he was right, as history proved.

He really liked Gene. He would often call Gene at the start of the work day since Gene was a calming influence. Gene was even asked to sit in for him in his large office while he was traveling in Japan. This was an honor, but it was a period of bomb scares which proved to be mostly fakes. Gene was praying that he would not be forced to make a decision to evacuate the facility.

That site manager eventually retired, and a replacement came to the site. On one occasion, Gene had a bout with the new site manager when he felt that the manager was being unfair. The manager changed his mind, but assigned Gene to a job as software quality manager. That was a stretch. An organic chemist in charge of software quality. He may have wanted Gene to fail and lose his top rating as an IBM employee. If so, that was his mistake.

When a particular software release was having some problems, Gene had to tell the site manager not to sign off on it for announcement. The producing group told Gene's staff that the manager was going to sign off this time, because the division president wanted it announced. At the review meeting, they gave a glowing presentation and thought that the announcement was cinched. At the finish of the presentation, the site manager turned to Gene with a smile and said, "Do I sign it now?" Gene said that if it were him, he would not sign it. Gene felt it had serious problems and would not pass muster. The site manager could not sign off with his quality manager disagreeing, especially if Gene was right. The meeting ended promptly.

As the saying goes, "There went his job" and career. Gene did have an offer as director of software quality for a Boston computer company, but he had turned it down. The company came back with a "money no object offer." He still turned it down. How they got his name, he did not know. A human resource person, who used to work for Gene, said he would have gained a small fortune if he had taken the opportunity to take his retirement pension and one year's pay, which IBM was offering to retirees, added to his new salary with the Boston company.

A day or two after the "Don't sign meeting," a software error was discovered in a customer's office field test. Gene was now a hero in his boss's eyes. If the site manager had approved the announcement and then had to pulled it back, he would be in trouble, especially if he had overruled the expert who was responsible for giving him advice. It was after that experience that Gene got his good management award, and yet another plaque.

His boss eventually got promoted to headquarters and he promoted Gene with him. This put Gene back in a headquarters position where he could match the money the sites were giving to universities for research contracts. It was Gene's old advance technology money shifted to this area.

Even when his boss left for another headquarters job, Gene was still his "go to guy." When a problem could not be solved by the normal routes, he called Gene. He called Gene when an IBM sales vice president could not get summer jobs and funding for female students at a college he was working with. Gene knew enough people with similar jobs who could get money for female students to work at the site. He got the promise of money and took care of convincing the site in question that they should agree to the positions. Gene did this all in one day. When Gene's former manager told the vice president who made the original request, the vice president was amazed that it had been done, and so quickly, since he could not get it done though the normal channel.

Gene in his inimitable style followed up later. The responsible site at that point had a freeze on summer hiring and was not going to fulfill the promise. Gene called the human resource director of the division and got him to agree that they should honor the promise. Problem solved. Neither his former manager nor the vice president knew of the snag that would have had the site renege on their promise.

Yet another time when IBM had trouble getting their computers on campus, Gene came up with the idea that in IBM's matching grants program they should offer more dollars towards their computers than the normal match as an option, perhaps a 3-1 match. The director of research, who had graduated with his PhD at an early age, told Gene that this was the most creative idea he had ever heard. Even though that was a spontaneous and obvious exaggeration, it floored Gene when he heard it. Gene's proposal was very successful in putting IBM computers on campuses.

Another example of Gene's creativity at IBM was when he helped the recruiting process by categorizing IBM jobs by skill, and produced a brochure very different from the glossy one containing little information that the recruiting arm had previously published. Now the students could talk about the actual job. IBM's recruiting success followed. The brochure was an attraction to get students to look at IBM for specific job descriptions and skills.

Gene was one of the senior managers to be selected to determine the validity of employee complaints which were sent to the top of IBM, and then to selected senior managers for investigation. He spent a lot of agonizing time at work, and home, to determine who was right. One of these was the firing of a mentally challenged employee. Gene discovered that part of the firing was for a violent action and after the firing there was a potentially dangerous action taken toward his manager.

He talked to the assistant of the CEO of IBM and suggested that it might be wise to do the interview by phone. All reviews and decisions in these matters were usually done face to face, in an IBM office, and the assistant refused. She said that if he was afraid, IBM security could be stationed outside the door in case things became threatening. Gene knew this was a useless suggestion, since the damage to him could be done before security could enter the room. He did not appreciate the afraid issue comment and as such decided to take the case. He flew on a day trip to California to meet with the employee. The interview went smoothly, but of course, this was only an information meeting and not a meeting which might cause the employee to react violently. Back at work, Gene received a call from his manager who had heard about the case and said that Gene did not have to take it. Gene said that he had already reviewed the case and was forming conclusions that would be reviewed at the corporate level, by the chairman's office. The head of the division was someone that Gene had had a prior disagreement with. In a somewhat revealing statement, the senior executive had mentioned to the human resource colleague that he was happy that Gene had the case, because he would deal with it with empathy.

Gene concluded that the firing was justified. He had been told that the employee could be given psychiatric help, at IBM's expense, and if he was cured of violent tendencies, could reapply to IBM. Corporate reviewed the conclusions and then called Gene telling him that the conclusions and the resulting offer were appropriate, and that he could conclude the review by phone with the employee, with his parents on the line. This not only bypassed the rule of face to face, but it allowed outsiders to hear the evidence. This was probably the first time this had been done in IBM history, and may have been the last time, because of the unusual circumstances. The call with the employee, and his parents, went very well. Gene and his colleagues were relieved.

I, of course, did not know all this was happening or I would have had a wifely disagreement. Did I say disagreement? It would have seemed like the wrath of Genghis Khan was descending, if I knew that Gene was possibly endangered.

After Gene retired from IBM, his technical work evolved into a consulting job helping Syracuse University obtain research grants.

The university appreciated Gene, but a couple of times they disagreed with him. They felt very strongly that their write-ups were sufficient and thought that he might agree with them. Gene held firm, noting that the approach they were taking in the proposal would not pass muster with technical experts. They finally used his approach and received a ten-million-dollar grant over ten years with a notation that it was the best presentation that the reviewing team had received. Another esteemed university used the approach that Gene had persuaded Syracuse to reject and failed to qualify for one of the grants available in that package.

Syracuse was ecstatic about Gene's help. Gene knew that it came naturally to him and felt he could have charged the university a much larger fee for his services. He used to read and mentally correct problems as they came off our fax machine. He would then sit down to more carefully review them. There were no additional charges. Gene was basing his figure on the time he spent to analyze the proposal and decide on a better way. Syracuse University in turn, based a somewhat higher figure on the value of the advice. The fee was still much lower than what other consultants would charge, but Gene did not care. The fact that his advice helped them is what mattered most. So much for my husband who was smart in some things, but not in realizing that the winning of a ten-million-dollar contract was worth more than the $800 he asked for. Syracuse boosted this amount to $1,000 dollars. I hesitate to say what other consultants would have charged, but they were both happy, and that mattered a lot to Gene.

The other grant on which Gene advised followed a similar path. The grant development officer objected strongly to Gene's comments, while acknowledging the fact that Gene also caught a chemical error. Gene finally prevailed and the contract was again cited by the reviewers as one of the best. He only charged $300 for that one since he only gave them common sense in strengthening the write-up. He received a call where he was asked to comment on a smaller proposal over the phone. Gene commented on it and when they asked him for the fee, he said that he would not charge anything for the call. A second call came shortly after the proposer had left the office and the development officer essentially told Gene that he was foolish in not charging a fee. Now, he did not say stupid, and I wouldn't say that either. Gene and that director remained friendly even after Gene stopped consulting in order to continue our coaching careers in Rhode Island and Massachusetts. I was naturally a big contributor to that decision.

One of the people who became friendly with Gene was John Karakash, the former Dean of Engineering at Lehigh University who was a consultant for IBM corporate vice presidents. He was known for his many quotable statements, which even Lee Iacocca the automobile executive had asked for. One of John's quotes even made the congressional record when a Michigan congressman was at the University of Michigan and heard John's talk. The part that he had inserted in the record was, "When I came to this country as an immigrant, they told me about the Bill of Rights. I wondered if there was a corresponding Bill of Responsibilities?" What a powerful quote. When he asked Gene to critique one of his future talks, I aided in the process. I also shopped for appropriate Christmas presents for him as that was not unusual for me. I bought presents for family, old friends, and other coaches that Gene volunteered for, as well as people at the school we coached at, including the president of the college. Wanting to buy Christmas presents for John, was part of my feeling that he was now part of our extended family.

I loved my girls and I enjoyed many a good time bringing them up to be ladies. Our oldest chose to attend Marist College in the town of Poughkeepsie on a Presidential scholarship which allowed her to take a large number of courses with recommended professors, and get her degree in three years. She was going to be a commuter so I decided that she should have her own car. My husband did not know much about fixing cars, so we bought a small new Datsun. After the first year, I decided that she should get to know dormitory life for full college appreciation. Gene used to say that it looked like a setup since we bought her a car and then we put her on campus. Now she has a car and campus life. In those days, that was a very good deal. To our surprise, when she got married shortly after graduation, she gave the car to her sister who was next in line for college. Erin and Kathleen both chose Johnson and Wales College in Rhode Island, so having cars was a requirement.

Shortly after the girls graduated from their respective colleges, they decided to get married. There I was now, not only dealing with graduations a few years apart, but also weddings. It was not only one of the busiest periods in my home life but, also one of my happiest. I loved to plan. Besides ensuring a great meal, I decided that since people had to drive home, that I would have sandwiches made for the latter part of the reception hoping that it would delay the effect of any alcohol they drank. It was unusual, but I wanted to ensure the guest's safety as much as I could in those days.

Mary Catherine, Erin, and Kathleen, married good men, Tom, Jim, and George, in that order, who treated Gene and me as if we were their own mother and father. Gene and I had the boys that we could not give birth to, along with three caring girls. The wall of happiness was reaching a peak. The girls were always part of our family council, helping to convince me how we could do things better. Gene would joke at times that he had four bosses; me and his three daughters. No one ever disagreed with that. I also teased the boys. One day I teased Jim, our most quiet son-in-law, and he gave me a teasing reply. I jokingly retorted that I liked him better when he was quiet. We both enjoyed ourselves with some ice breaking. Our family enlarged, not only with the girl's husband's families, but it also brought us seven grandchildren (Kimberly, Christopher, Amy, Matthew, Andrew, Kasey, and Hanna) and seven great grandchildren (Madeline, Penelopy, Abigail, Logan, Archer, Hunter, and Stella). I was in my glory with so many children to spoil. It was the perfect job for me, and what more could one ask for.

In The Eyes of an Alzheimer's Patient

Gene Damm

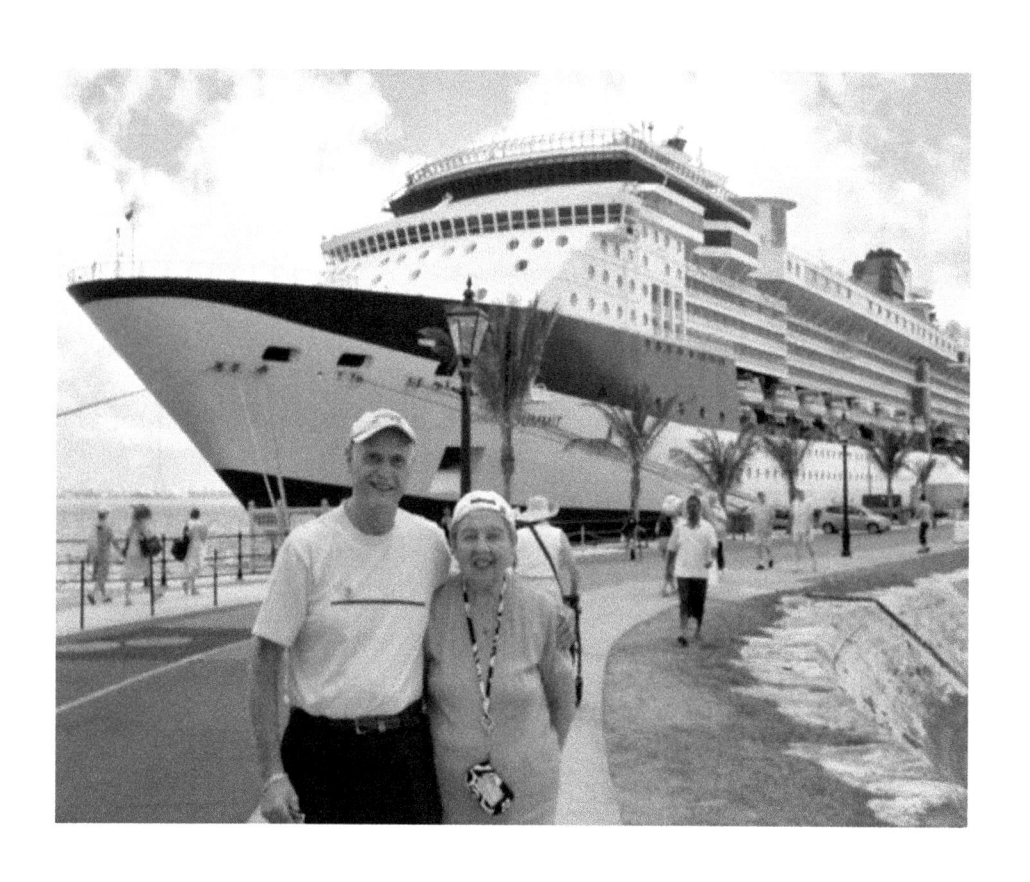

Some of Our Travels

The title is a little deceiving as they were really mostly vacations for me and the girls, while Gene worked at that location. Once when we lived in Endicott, Gene had to give a presentation to the National Security Agency at Fort Meade near Washington DC. All the clearances were received and he gave his talk on a project that he was working on. He wanted me to go with him and I thought that it would also be good for the girls. However, I would only go if we could take our babysitter. So, there was Gene in a facility with armed servicemen while I and my entourage were having a ball touring the Washington DC area in one of those chartered limousines. After his presentation, we drove back to Endicott. It was years later when we took my father to see the Capitol that Gene finally got to enjoy the sites.

Another trip to DC worth mentioning was when Gene was on a committee to try to persuade math majors to major in computer science. He was amazed that the person representing the Bureau of Labor Statistics was so fascinated by his presentation since a lot of the statistics he presented were from the bureau's own database. In later years, he felt that the committees focus on math majors was a mistake since computer science would grow on its own and that the country still needed pure and applied math majors in their own right.

Gene Damm

I traveled with Gene to a number of places, sometimes reluctantly. Once he had a hard time convincing me to go to Chicago with him where he had a meeting. I agreed at the last minute and Gene canceled his flight. We packed up the girls and took the train. The only thing was that he originally did not have a large enough room for the five of us. When we got to Chicago, we tried to change the room, but it was convention time and they were turning people away that did not have reservations. They said that they did not have a suitable room for five so Gene insisted that we could make the smaller room work with cots. The hotel insisted that it was impossible. After a while they decided to put us in a large double room suite and gave the girls several gifts while holding the low price that IBM had contracted for. Gene later talked to the manager of the hotel to see if we should pay more, but the manager would hear none of it. The girls and I took the bus to tour Chicago and attended the famous Kungsholm Puppet Opera theater there. People on the bus in Chicago were very pleasant to me and the girls, which was nice to see in a big city. Our family ate dinner together at one of Chicago's steak houses near the hotel, and when the girls were asked the next day where they wanted to eat, they opted to go back to the same restaurant. The hostess had mispronounced our last name when announcing the table and the girls had corrected her. The next day, the hostess pronounced it correctly. Even though she was not the person taking the reservation, but remembered despite the large number of people eating there. We were very impressed.

When the meeting ended, we took the train directly home. I enjoyed all the trips we made together even though Gene had to work while the girls and I were enjoying ourselves. The main thing was that Gene would return home after a normal day and this approach kept the family together. The wall of happiness was still rising.

We had our 50th Wedding Anniversary at a reception facility when we could not take the family on a cruise with us due to the conflict of the children's high school and college vacations. My granddaughter Kimberly was the Mistress of Ceremonies. During her talk, she mentioned that her grandfather taught her that "practice does not make perfect, but perfect practice does." Then she mentioned that her grandmother taught her that you will have to kiss a lot of frogs before you meet your prince. I was so pleased that she remembered what I had told her when she and a boyfriend parted ways in high school. She had now met her prince and he was at the ceremony. I also configured a trivia game based on histories of the 1950's. One of my daughters thought that it was too corny, but I ignored the warning. I was like that. We offered a prize for the people who filled in the most correct answers and our guests loved it. It became so competitive that one of the middle age guests called his mother to try to get one of the answers.

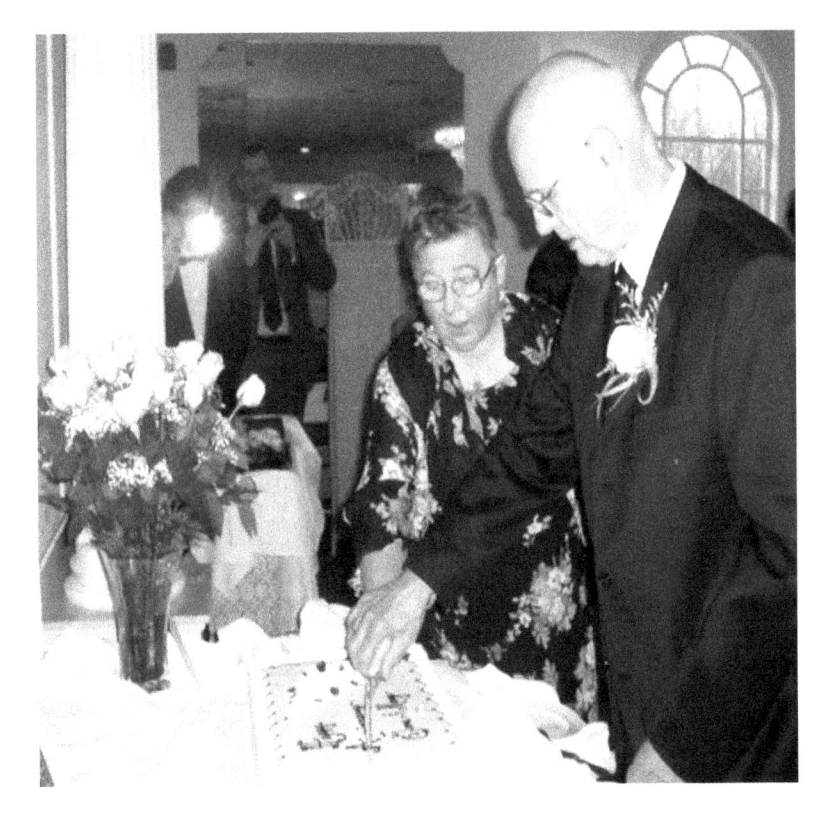

At the reception, there were the parents of two of our lesson swimmers who traveled from the Boston area to attend the ceremony. The two wives were dancing a very fast dance and Gene joined them. He then danced several other similar dances with them to the amazement of one of the husbands. Do you think that this was very smart for a man in his early seventies, who had two prior heart attacks? I will let you answer that since I do not want to comment. You already know what it would be. He obviously survived, but that does not change the sanity of it.

Gene and I did take some pleasure trips for ourselves when the girls were all married. These included trips to Europe. Kathleen once asked why we didn't do this when they were younger. The answer was simple. We could not afford it with bringing up three girls, while paying for three college tuition's and three weddings.

Our trips to Europe consisted primarily tours of England, Scotland, and Ireland, Gene and I both loved Ireland with the thatched roofs and the view of the cliffs of Mohr, which can reach as high as 702 feet above sea level with massively high waves bouncing off them. They are awesome. The people both there and in England were very friendly. Gene and I completely enjoyed the historical sites in London, and the folk lore in the Scottish Highlands.

In one of our visits to England we were able to see my cousin who still lived in Preston where my mother was born. When we were visiting my cousin for a day, she asked if we wanted to go pub crawling. It took us awhile to realize it meant bar hopping. It was a delightful experience. The people were very social and it was almost like watching the John Wane movie "The Quiet Man". The people welcomed us and you could see them spinning yarns about local happenings. It seemed like we were thrown back in time.

Our most memorable cruise was to Alaska watching the iridescent blue of the partially submerged icebergs. We loved learning the local lore such as that many people had to get their water from cisterns during their dry season and that in the remote areas there may not be a full-time doctor. What a difference from our trip to Hawaii. In Hawaii there was ample water and medical help, and on a snorkeling cruise to Molokini crater we saw more whales than you could imagine.

My favorite vacation spot was Cape Cod. We could easily reach our hometown of New Bedford and tour their new and extensive whaling museum and eat at a wonderful Portuguese restaurant called Antonio's. I loved to shop at the various Christmas Tree Shops there and visit the glass museums. My favorite was the Sydenstricker Glass Gallery & Workshop, where I could buy beautiful glass dishes for family and close friends, as well as myself. And of course, get filled up with my favorite treat of homemade ice cream. One of the places we frequented made individual waffle cones on the spot. Yummy! A real fresh waffle cone filled with your favorite homemade ice cream. I would be remiss if I did not mention that we got our fill of fish and chips and stuffed quahogs at a fish shack, called Gene's of all things, on the bridge between New Bedford and Fairhaven, during many of our annual trips. My oldest daughter's mother-in-law would accompany us at one of our two timeshares there.

Gene Damm

A Difficult Decision

During Gene's career at IBM, I was taking care of our girls and also dealing with elderly parents. My mother was having eating problems, possibly because of her oncoming dementia. My father, like a lot of husbands in that situation, could not convince her to eat. We made frequent four-hour trips to New Bedford, Massachusetts to encourage her appetite only to find that all of these were short term fixes. We ultimately brought my parents to live with us in Poughkeepsie, which impacted our family life. The girls had their lives changed dramatically. We had to deal with the various health and personal issues associated with aging parents. If I suggested that we all go out for a ride and my parents refused, no one went. One time when the girls were in college, we went to a swim meet and did leave them at home for the day. I suggested that we start a fire in our fireplace to make it cozier for them. Gene lit the fire, but did not realize that the flue was closed. When we arrived home, we found them huddled in a side room and the house filled with smoke. We asked them why they did not call the fire department, but they did not give a good answer. Talk about feeling guilty. I guess it could have been worse.

My mother's dementia was also getting worse. At night she would thrash in bed so badly that it became a dangerous situation and I had to restrain her with sheets so that she would not fall off the bed. After that she had to be put in the hospital and our family doctor told me that I could not take care of her at home anymore. This time was extremely difficult. Little did I realize that I would eventually develop dementia also and my dear husband would have to deal with it.

We decided to put my mother in a nursing home where a friend of ours worked. She had good care and my friend gave her back rubs to alleviate the bed sores she acquired in the hospital. She only survived for three more weeks.

After my mother passed away, we took my father with us on our out of town meets. He was a frail person at that time and it seemed to be the best solution rather than leaving him at home. That created problems when he hurt his knee while Gene was helping him down the stairs on our way to a meet. We had a nurse on the team check him out as the pain lingered. She thought he sprained his knee. However, since the pain was still there when we got home, we had it further checked out and found that it was fractured. Another time, I thought that he would enjoy sitting outside on the patio at our hotel room to get some fresh air. He must have stared at the sun too long and damaged his eye. So much for trying to be helpful.

He also had a severe bleeding ulcer and did not want to eat while at the hospital. When we visited him there, we saw several full protein shakes on the table. A nurse clued me in that one of the doctors had suggested that they "pull the plug on him." I was furious and took steps to let people know that I was not consulted and would not agree to it. When he got home, I encouraged him to eat, but I found him feeding his food to the dog or hiding it in a napkin. I then resorted to making my own milkshakes which included ice cream and other useful nutrients. He did get some nourishment and improved.

My father fell when we were on vacation in a town near New Bedford, Massachusetts, and injured his hip. We took him to the small hospital there where they operated. Unfortunately, they were not able to restore it, and he needed a second operation. The surgeon was very nice and thoughtful. He even came in on his day off to visit him and me. I spent a lot of time at the hospital with my father, and the doctor was very comforting.

To make matters worse, about the time that my father was admitted to the hospital, Gene became very ill. I stayed in town to watch over my father while he was in the hospital. Our oldest daughter, Mary, and her family took Gene back to Poughkeepsie to see our primary doctor. He had the symptoms of mononucleosis, but our doctor thought that he was too old for that, even though he was getting fevers of 104 degrees and was very weak. We talked over the phone and he was trying to cover up his squeaky voice and sickness, but to no avail. He did not want me to worry about him while I was worrying about my father.

Gene was staying at Mary's and her husband Tom's house when the call came in that my father had passed away. The surgeon had attempted a second operation on my father's knee because of the complications from the first surgery, but he was too weak to survive. Our doctor then put Gene in the hospital in Poughkeepsie to enable the family to attend the funeral in Massachusetts. Unfortunately, Gene could not attend his father-in-law's funeral due to his health. While Gene was in the hospital, it was confirmed that he did actually have mononucleosis. He had also acquired hepatitis, causing the hospital to put him in a private room. This was a precaution as it did not appear to be contagious. He recovered and life went on.

In The Eyes of an Alzheimer's Patient

Gene Damm

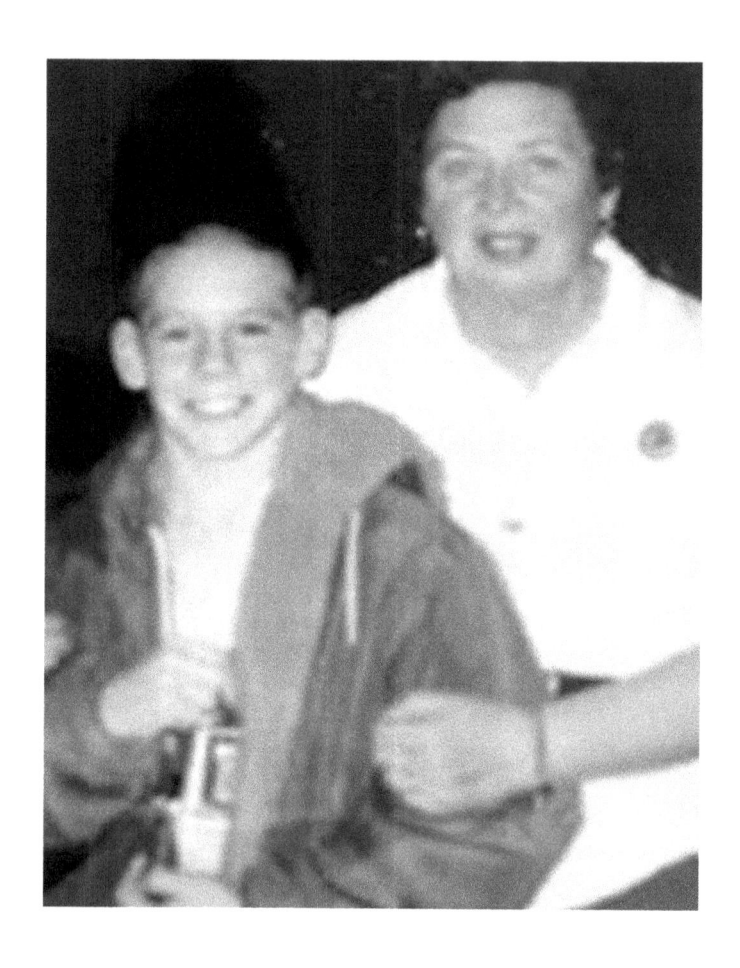

Mary and One of the Swimmers Who Became Top16 in the Nation in his Stroke

In The Eyes of an Alzheimer's Patient

Our Coaching Careers

We loved to do volunteer work and one that I volunteered for was through our church. It involved heading up the youth program and helping with a swim team sponsored by the Catholic Youth Organization (CYO) to prepare the swimmers for their annual summer meet. Naturally, our girls were on the team, and we decided to make it a year-round team. Guess who played the major role in that decision with us coaching it? The "we," was me. I decided, but Gene and I did it together. Coming from New Bedford, Massachusetts, which was known as the whaling city, it was an easy choice for me to name the team the Saint Mary's Whalemen.

Even with minimal water time, the team flourished. Making it a year-round team proved to be the right decision. Our swimmers achieved top sixteen rankings in their national age group. One of our swimmers ranked number one in the nation in his age group for the backstroke, along with high rankings in his other strokes. When he was at a USA swim meet for swimmers in the northeast of the country, he swam five individual events and won all five. He achieved a junior national qualifying time at the young age of thirteen. The Junior National meet was at Fort Lauderdale, Florida and this was when I decided to fly there to watch our swimmer compete. Prior to that, when the girls were young and my parents were alive, I would only take trains when we traveled alone or as a family. It turned out that I liked flying. We then flew together to Junior National meets after that. Gene did fly to a Senior National meet by himself when it occurred at the same time that we were hosting a meet, and I stayed back to coach the rest of the team.

Keep in mind that none of this success would have been possible if I had not volunteered us to take on this responsibility. I came up with the idea, and although Gene blossomed in the role, initially he was playing "Follow the Leader." Gene became a successful coach, and I soon assumed a subordinate role as his assistant coach. In his coaching career, Gene coached mostly by teaching and motivating, not yelling and criticizing. We were both successful in our roles. He was a motivator and I was a disciplinarian. That was another way that we were different and complimentary. The key was that we both loved children and they loved us despite our different approaches. At camps, when I took my ten-year-old swimmers to the cafeteria, they were told that they could talk as much as they wanted on the way there, but they were not to talk on the way back. Instead, they were to concentrate on what they learned in the morning so that they could execute it in the afternoon. We alternated pool time with dry-land instruction, so each one of us had the pool to ourselves.

Gene always had a thirst for knowledge and worked diligently to pass that on to others. He followed up on current thinking, but drew his own opinions on what would work. He tried to understand not just the swimming strokes, but also the mechanism by which they worked. Therefore, he had new ideas of his own. When we wrote our first swimming book, the editor of Swimming World Magazine, who published it, said that it was the first time he had seen the use of the core of the body in swimming put into print. Today everybody talks about the use of the core. Gene recognizing the role of the core by his study of the martial arts. He may not have been the first to recognize it, but we were one of the first to put it in a publication. At one point, Gene mentioned the concept to a former Olympian who appeared to slough it off. A few years later, when it became a popular theme, that former Olympian became a strong advocate for it. I, of course, was the co-author of the publication and focused on what young beginning swimmers needed to know to succeed. With all his success in coaching, Gene still feels that he talks about his achievements primarily because of his inferiority complex that I was never able to help him to conquer. At a later stage, we became one of the first coaches to recognize the value of a swimmer keeping their head in line with their body. At that time, many swimmers carried their heads higher in freestyle. Gene had read about a recreation coach in England using a technique where his swimmers heads were more in line with their body. We were unable to meet with the coach when we were in England, but Gene thought that it made good sense, so we implemented it. Some of our lesson swimmers said their coach was critical of the technique, until Swimming World Magazine published an article stating that the Australians had also come to the same conclusion.

In our early days of coaching, we had a ten and under relay team which was close to being submitted for top ten in the nation in the medley relay. Gene told them that if they were ever going to make the team, it had to be that day, since the butterfly swimmer was going to age up and she was a key swimmer for them. With that motivation, they went from not being considered for submission into being ranked number two in the nation. We even took on a swimmer with attention deficit syndrome and poor times. Gene worked with his stroke and mindset, and within two years, he scored in the first Junior National meet that he had qualified for. That was not unique. We were able to take on weaker swimmers and bring them to a national status, even with the minimal pool time that was available to us.

One of our neighbors of Chinese descent had children on the team. They were wonderful to us and their children were almost like our own. We ate a lot of great Chinese food, thanks to their generosity. One time, one of the boys dropped over egg rolls because his mother made a "few extra." There sat about twenty on the plate. Our daughters liked their rice dishes so much, that when Theresa Chu asked what she could help with for the weddings, Kathleen asked her for her rice dish for the head table. We were a little embarrassed, but Kathleen loved the dish. On her wedding day there was a big rice bowl at the head table to go with the prime rib meal. We were once included at a lunch for special friends before their daughter's wedding. We had the soup first, and pretty much our fill at the next serving, only to realize that it was an eleven course Chinese banquet. Boy, we were filled that day. At one of their son's weddings in Manassas, Virginia, we were again invited to a dinner for special friends the night before the wedding. This time we realized that it was another eleven course banquet and ate more leisurely.

The team loved the Chu children. At one League championship Bonnie Chu was in a mixed age group relay with her brothers and another girl. The girl made up a sheet for the relay to win saying, "Chugga, Chu, Chu, Chu." Normally we would put the fastest swimmer at the end of the relay, but this time we put Bonnie Chu last even though she was the youngest. The rest of the relay team knew that they would have to give Bonnie a lot of room in the pool. They won with Bonnie swimming the time of her life against an older and faster male swimmer. It made for a lot of cheering in the final leg of the race as the distance between the two swimmers tightened.

Our powerhouse Catholic Youth Organization (CYO) team had increased in strength and admiration, but we also made room for a down syndrome girl. I played a large roll in this. The team loved Mary. We were at a dual meet when she had aged up from the ten and under age group to the 11-12 age group. I still wanted to put her in a decent relay, so I moved up three of the fast ten-year-old girls to swim the relay with her, which you could do under the rules. They came in second and one of the most wonderful things happened. One of the girls on the relay came up to me and said that they had lost the relay, but they had three ten-year-old girls swimming against the 11-12 year old's. That is a teaching lesson for adults when they hear it. Prejudices, along with biases, are not basic to children. They are learned.

Gene still feels that there should be scholarships for down syndrome and autistic children to participate on competitive teams. Their abilities may surprise people through skill and social development, if properly trained, as some teams have recognized. Better still, how about a year-round team for children with challenges where the team was obligated to move a swimmer up to a mainstream team if they improved to a competitive level. Coaches from local teams could help make that decision, while they were guest coaching. Think about that. Many children on the autism spectrum are brilliant beyond belief, but have difficulty socializing. This would be a great opportunity to enhance their development with their peers.

For a while we had a swimmer from France on the team while his father was on assignment in Poughkeepsie, New York for IBM. Under Gene's tutelage, the swimmer achieved a backstroke time that would have been a top time in France for his age. There we were, with the top backstroke swimmer for France and the number one in our country for their age groups. At a championship meet, they both beat the former world record holder and Olympic champion in backstroke in a preliminary event. The former world record holder was not in top shape at the time, but still with the go and pride of a champion, he came over to talk with Gene. He said that he would hate to lose to kids as young as these. Gene's response to him was, "Just take it out on them." Gene meant that he should start out faster than them, and then keep it going. Great swimmers know how to take it out and maintain the pace with almost every ounce of energy. He won by a fair margin, but it was quite a day for our swimmers. A similar situation occurred at another time with another former Olympian where our swimmer had beat him with his famous underwater kick in the preliminary heat. Needless to say, the final outcome was the same. Race strategy is very important, but most athletes do not really expend their maximum energy, but great athletes come closer to it.

Gene Damm

We wanted all our swimmers to challenge themselves regardless of the competition so that they were ready for the final completion of the season. A great acting performance on stage requires great rehearsals. It is the same way with athletes.

The team was like family to us and after meets many of them would go to a restaurant for pizza with us. We also shared picnics and other events. One time at a team softball competition, as a fun thing for the team, Gene was on one of the sides opposite a high school softball pitcher who was also on our swim team. She threw one in close to Gene his first time at bat and he faked falling down as if he was hit. It was his joke, but she felt so bad at the possibly of hitting her coach that she threw softer pitches to him next time. Armed with a metal bat, that man who'd been an awkward athlete in his youth, had been the hero of his side.

We did not command respect locally in the early days of our volunteer coaching, even though our younger swimmers were some of the best around. Being volunteer coaches did a lot to create the image of not being as good as paid coach. We were more respected outside our area as they looked at the results, not the pay scale. Eventually that changed locally as our older swimmers qualified for national meets with the resulting publicity of their accomplishments. Our team had far exceeded anyone's expectations. The 17–18 year old 400 yard freestyle relay team that broke the Junior national relay record and became the number one in the nation for that event helped to change the image locally.

While still at IBM, Gene used a lot of his vacation days for swim meets. He had a lot of them in the bank and did not mind using them that way. He never asked for a community service day which he could have. Gene sometimes worked a half day, but submitted a full day of vacation, even though it would have been allowed to claim only a half day vacation or not come to work at all that day. One of the swimmers told his mother that he would like to have a job like Gene's because he was never there. Little did he know.

In The Eyes of an Alzheimer's Patient

We traveled to meets and stayed at hotels at our own expense during our time with the CYO team. With Gene working and me taking care of my mom and dad along with our coaching, my husband and I were spread thin, and it was about to get even thinner.

Gene by now had a weakness for helping people, even with our crowded schedule. A master's team needed a coach and he volunteered to help them. So much for teaching him to volunteer. I had created a monster waiting to attack his health, and neither one of us realized where the cut off point for him was. We were having fun.

I volunteered Gene for many coaching jobs including one with his first college team. Vassar College had initially asked me if I wanted the job, but I felt that Gene had more coaching skills. I convinced him to be their head coach. I bet nobody knows that I was offered the job first.

I was happy that Gene would have that opportunity, and that was all that mattered. The team performed so well the first year that the athletic director asked Gene what he wanted for the team. Gene chose a large record board. He felt that if the team saw the existing records that there would be incentive to break them, and they did. A number of those new records existed long after Gene had moved on. The following year, at the urging of the assistant coach who was an instructor at the college and knew the athletic director well, came the acquisition and installation of the electronic timing system. They were now looking like a college with a serious swim team. Gene had wanted to have the record board, in order for the swimmers to have goals. As a result, a number of prior records were broken.

When our minimal pool time was further reduced for our age group team, Gene was able to get the top swimmers more pool time at Vassar College on Saturday morning. However, in order to not overtly impact the college, only our better swimmers had an extra practice. To us it was frustrating not being able to give the whole team that opportunity. We were a family, as well as a team.

Gene Damm

At one point in time, I was helping to coach a high school team with a parent of one of our swimmers. The requirement was that the head coach had to be a teacher in the school system, and when nobody stepped up for the job, she agreed to take the job with me being her assistant. I took the less experienced swimmers and made them competitive. Some of those swimmers even moved on to the division championships. After the high school practice, Gene and I joined up at the college pool where he coached and had a sandwich together, before we went to our age group practice.

For a short time, I was also a partner in a store that sold swimming and ballet accessories called, "On Your Toes." I am very good at making up names. I was not only one of the sales people, but I also carefully kept the books to ensure that we accounted for everything, which was very helpful at tax time. While Gene and I did not have much time for ourselves, the wall of happiness was still being built even higher, with the joy that came from all these activities. I did sell my share of the store to my partner after a few years.

Another New Adventure

Eventually, we accepted jobs as swim coaches for an age group team at The United States Military Academy at West Point. Gene had earlier rejected an offer from them, even though they were paid positions. We were still reluctant to accept this offer, but were convinced to take the job by one of our fellow coaches on another team. We had more pool time, specifically two hours of pool time, five days a week. It was a big increase in pool time, even though less than a lot of teams on the national scene. The downside was that he had to give up his college coaching job.

It was a much longer commute for us, especially for Gene, since it meant commuting even further from Kingston, New York, where he worked at the time. Some of our swimmers followed us even with the longer commuting distance. One family, who lived across the river from Kingston, was gracious enough to feed Gene when he stopped by to the pick up their swimmer to take him to practice. The boy's father picked the boy up in Poughkeepsie, after practice, for the trip further north to his home. Both were nice gestures and showed their appreciation for Gene's efforts. That swimmer ended up being the Captain of the Ohio State swim team.

This new engagement paid dividends for both us and the swimmers. It was there that we developed a 17-18 age group relay team which not only won at Junior Nationals, but broke a record that was held for a number of years until the meet's highest age qualification was raised to 19, which allowed college age swimmers to compete. It was also the number one ranked swim team in the country, for the 17-18 age group in the 400-yard freestyle relay that year. Getting college scholarships for three of our swimmers, who were in their senior year was relatively easy. One swimmer wanted to go to Penn State and was offered a modest scholarship. Early one morning, Gene was called by the coach's wife, who was a former Olympian, to say her husband was so impressed by the swimmer's performance that he was increasing the offer. However, while coming out of a meet, Gene was walking next to the Syracuse University coach and asked him why he did not offer that swimmer a scholarship. The coach said that it was because his scholarship funds for the year were exhausted. Soon after that, the Syracuse coach called the swimmer offering a full scholarship. The mother of the boy then called Gene to see what they should do. Gene indicated that since the boy really wanted to go to Penn State, that they should send him there. If they could not afford the difference, then they would have to talk to their son. The swimmer went to Penn State and became a team captain and an All American. He now coaches a high school team where he teaches.

Gene worked hard to get scholarships for his swimmers. He worked tirelessly to get whatever money he could get and we paid our own telephone bills to make this happen. When he heard that one college coach had backed off from her original position of a full scholarship, to a half scholarship for one of our female swimmers, he immediately called the coach and reminded her of what she had said earlier. She told Gene that she had split the final offer with another swimmer the she also wanted. That fell on deaf ears and Gene asked her what she was going to do about it. Possibly because she wanted future swimmers from us, she went back to her athletic director and got extra money from his budget.

Gene was then given a level 5 ranking in the American Swimming Association. It was the highest level one could achieve. At the time he received it, he was one of about 300 coaches who had reached that level nationally. He was also given it for age group coaching and was one of only a dozen or so coaches holding both honors. I in turn was coaching the younger swimmers, as well as coordinating the individual entries of our swimmers in the various meet events. It was not a trivial job and took a lot of work. The whole coaching effort exemplified the team of Gene and Mary. In all of this, he was able to maintain his number one ranking in IBM as one of their most valuable employees.

When he attended a retirement luncheon for a corporate vice president, he heard the VP say to the CEO of IBM that Gene was one of the best employees in IBM. Gene appreciated that, but knew that the compliment and one dollar would only buy him a cup of coffee.

In coaching, Gene had the recognition he deserved. I was his assistant coach, but he knew that I was an important person in developing our younger swimmers' talents and their zest for competitive swimming. His job was to fine tune their strokes for higher levels of competition. He used to tell people that great swimmers had great training from their early coaches. The team also recognized that I was an important cog in the work that I did, not only in coaching, but also setting up meet rosters and meet entries, and they rewarded me for it.

An example of our former swimmer's success became apparent when we had the men's team captain at Penn State and Ohio State as well as the women's team captain at Maine. We were ecstatic. It was the team of Gene and Mary that produced great swimmers. One of our former swimmer's parents remarked to the effect, that we were a perfect combination. Me with my disciplinary, yet loving approach, and Gene with his motivational and coaching skills. These attributes, which were much like an artist, were what made us a success and we never changed that approach.

One of the boys far exceeded his own expectations. Before we took over the new team, he had told his mother that he would never make a national time. He not only achieved Junior national, but also

Senior National times. He went on to make All American status in college. I used to feel bad that Gene did not get credit for the swimmers he had competing on high school teams. He told me not to worry about it because the swimmers and the parents knew. One of our swimmers, after achieving national acclaim told the press that he owed his success to his age group coach, Gene Damm. My husband was now vindicated from my concern of lack of public recognition for his achievement. That's my husband. Sometimes I felt that he did not push himself enough, and that was certainly true in IBM, but in this case, he was right in taking the higher road.

Another boy qualified for Olympic trials in his final college meet. He had originally left the first college where he had been offered a scholarship when they had a change in coaching staff. Gene tried hard to convince him to stay if he liked the school. His grades suffered and he finally left. Gene said that he would only train him if he agreed to go back to a college, assuming that they could find one to complete his degree. The boy accepted that and Gene worked hard to find a new school for him. He finally got him a good scholarship at another school where he made Division 1 All American status and also achieved an Olympic trial qualifying time.

The one thing that Gene did not like was that the age group team we had taken over at the United States Military Academy had a most valuable swimming award which was usually given to the best swimmer. Gene felt that if the fastest swimmer was automatically given the award, it would have looked like favoritism for the fastest swimmer. There appeared to be no way to satisfy all the parents, especially if they felt that their swimmer deserved to be recognized.

He avoided controversy by picking an average swimmer who had helped taking the lane ropes in and out of the pool and who voluntarily helped with the younger swimmers during meets. Gene truly believed that it was the right decision. When he announced that decision, everyone thought that it was a great decision when he explained it. A break from tradition which turned out well and would be food for thought for other teams who had that award to consider.

By the way, the fastest swimmer was very modest. In his younger years he held a number one in the nation ranking for backstroke and top 16 in the nation for other events. With all his modesty, he was elected captain of the Ohio State swim team in his junior and senior years.

The year that our men's team won the 400-yard freestyle relay and achieved the number one team in that event for the country, it was against teams with more pool time and money to pay for it. It was quite a sight to see our team on the top point of the awards podium wearing shorts and not the dressy uniforms other top finalist wore. Gene was rewarded with a framed certificate signed by the base commandant. Both of us had received several awards throughout our swimming careers, but this one was exceptional.

Gene's IBM managers recognized his ability to coach, as well as his technical and management skills, even though he took a lot of vacation days to attend meets. Once he reluctantly agreed to give a presentation when his manager agreed to put him on first, so he could finish early and drive to Fordham University for the start of a championship meet. In the meantime, I and his assistant coach would cover the swimmers until he got there.

He was wound up in his presentation and enjoying it, when his manager suddenly said, "We have heard enough." Gene was confused, since he thought the presentation was going very well. Then his manager added, "I will tell you the real reason we wanted you to be here." He then gave Gene a check for $5,000 and a plaque for good management. His manager then turned to the division president, who was also a corporate vice-president, and said, "Gene has to go now. He has a swim meet." Talk about being on top of the wall of happiness. He arrived at the swim meet in a business suit and was the best dressed coach there. He may have looked strange, but he was not going to miss some coaching by taking the time to change. Wow, I was so proud of him.

Gene Damm

A Major Change in the Road

Gene eventually had his first heart attack. No wonder! Getting up at 5:30 a.m. to travel back and forth, five days a week, to work in White Plains had finally caught up with him at age 57. The travel of up to sixty miles one way, plus traveling to go to practice and swim meets miles away for years, along with eating late dinners did not help his well-being. Gene still desired to return to coaching after that and our family council agreed that this would be good for him. While I was worried about his health, I could not argue with the family council that emotionally this would be good for him. This bump in the road was not going to stop us. I really worried whether this was the right decision. When things worked out so well, I reversed fields and I was the one who encouraged him to go back to coaching after some other serious incidents.

We were one, and while we were divided in our responsibilities and even some likes and dislikes, he usually caved in to me knowing that it was in his best interest. For example, when I convinced him that we needed to take breaks from swimming between seasons to the benefit of both us and the swimmers. Gene had plenty of vacation left after using some of it for swimming meets during the year, so we did get some vacations. He still had quite a few left over when he retired which he took advantage of in the way of financial compensation. You could do that in those days. The decision of the family that he should return to full coaching as well as working at IBM, was not one I would have agreed to if I did not have the benefit of their advice.

Gene finally retired from IBM, after I suggested (polite word) that he should either give up IBM or his coaching. IBM was in the process of downsizing and Gene did not want to release people he would have to if a quota was applied to his area. That was not his style, so he agreed with me and put in for retirement, which at the time would give you one year extra pay if you retired.

Even though the IBM pension was a lower percentage of his salary than what many other employers offered, he had reduced it to ensure a better standard of living for me. He was still the major source of income for the family along with our coaching salaries, we were still able to live comfortably. They then offered him a six-month package, at his normal pay, if he stayed on longer for the transition of his job. What a deal. It sure helped that first year, since it added substantially to our coaching salaries.

Gene's retirement luncheon was attended by a number of IBM corporate vice presidents, along with his personal friends and family. Many people, including the corporate vice presidents, wrote glowing reviews of him which were printed in a book that they presented to him. That part of his life was over. He now had only one career.

We were still living a hectic life, but it was extremely enjoyable. He was the acknowledged boss in coaching. I was still the boss when it came to the family. He'd had an unbelievable reversal in his work and coaching responsibilities, but in our marriage, he reverted to his subservient personality, another thing he never could totally conquer.

In addition to all we were doing, I volunteered Gene for everything, including rides to help people in need to give help to others.

Gene Damm

Some of this Gene did not really appreciate, but I had already offered it, so he did it.

With all of this, we were still on top of that wall of happiness. I had played a major role in getting him into coaching which helped him to follow his overwhelming desire to teach.

Like teenagers who feel they are indestructible, we had no idea that something like Alzheimer's would make our wall of happiness fall. With Gene's early heart attacks, he always thought that he would pass away before me, until my Alzheimer's got really bad. Later on, he prayed that he would hang on so that he could be my caregiver and I did not have to be put in a nursing home.

In The Eyes of an Alzheimer's Patient

Gene Damm

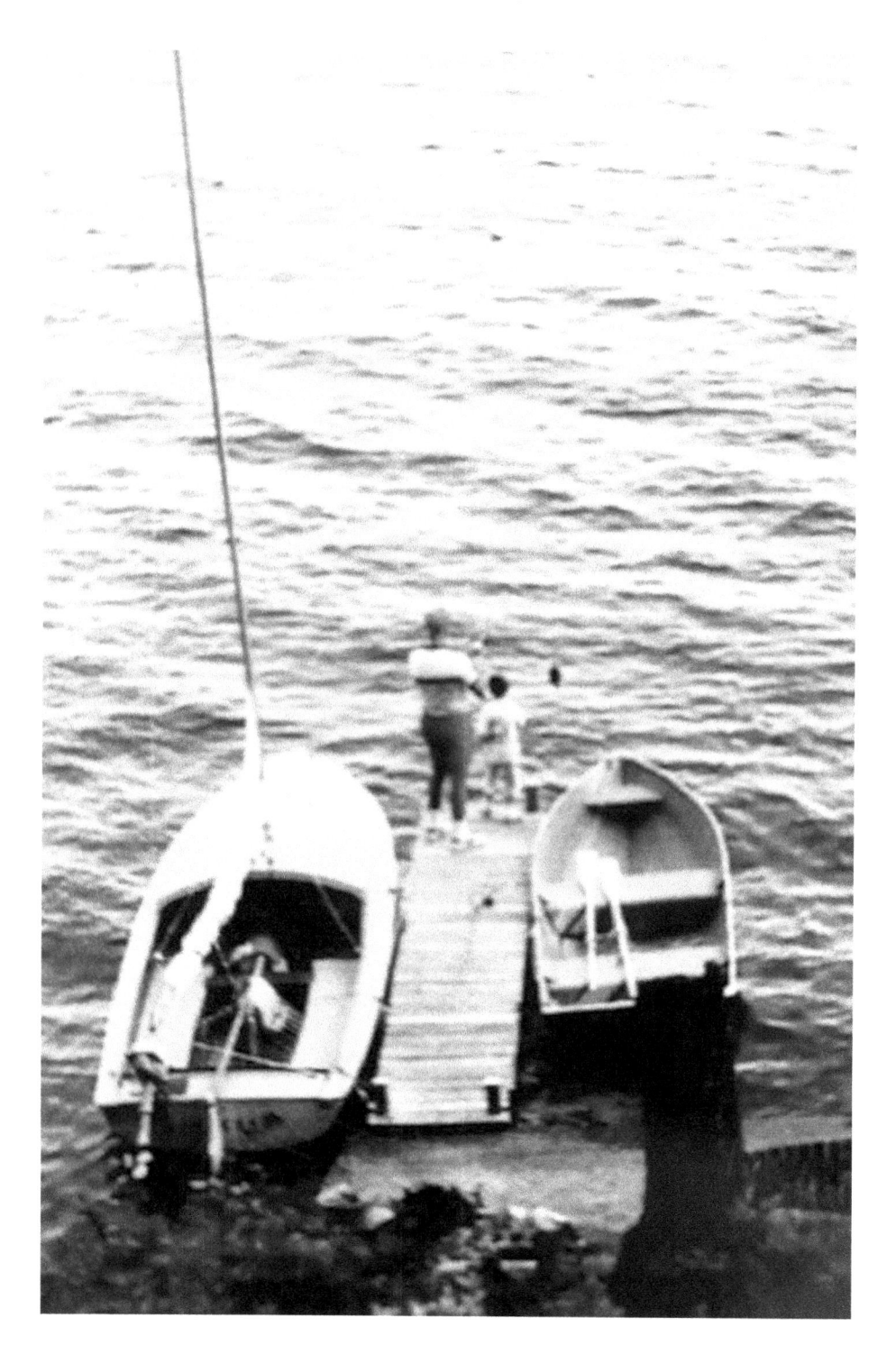

In The Eyes of an Alzheimer's Patient

Life at the Cottage

Our next adventure was when we moved to coach in the New England area, reasonably close to where we were born. We lived on Long Pond, a lake in a suburb of New Bedford, in a cottage we had bought a few years back. It was an old cottage with a small eating area, two bedrooms, a bath, and a cellar, which held the furnace and washing machine. The cellar was only accessed from the exterior of the cottage. The cottage was located on a hill overlooking the lake. We had a large deck built with stairs down to the lake. Our son-in-law Tom built twin piers so that he could dock our bowrider speedboat, our rowboat, as well as his sailboat. The speedboat was not used much except when company was there. Gene preferred the rowboat with an outboard motor which he could maneuver across the lake to preferred fishing areas. Fishing was his real love when we were there.

Unfortunately, with the time constraints of coaching and traveling to practice and meets, Gene was not able to fish as much as he would have liked. Regardless, the cottage made a good base of operation. We were thinking of renting our house in New York, but then Gene had another illness and I decided that a man who had so many things that could go wrong, along with the uncertainty of any move, that we should not rent it out. Gene, of course, did not argue with me, even though the house would remain empty for an unknown period of time. These things did not bother him as long as we were happy. The expenses of keeping an empty house in the Northeast did not bother me, and Gene did not care about the lost income as much as he did not want to contest my decision.

We initially took coaching positions with a team in Rhode Island. Gene was head coach of the senior team, which he coached at a different pool than the younger swimmers. Gene would take me to the pool I was helping at and then go to his pool miles away, returning to pick me up after practice was over. I worked under the coach of the younger swimmers. I made a mistake in criticizing something the younger team coach was doing and expressing it in front of a board member who apparently was not a fan of that coach. At one of the upcoming board meetings, the member mentioned something about the coach and I spoke up defending the coach. The board member was confounded. He later talked to Gene telling him that he had the coach in a weak position and I botched his efforts. Gene told the member that the man really didn't understand me. If something was wrong in my mind, I had no reservations about saying it. I also had no reservations if I felt a person was being unfairly accused of stating that either.

Once, Gene and I traveled a number of miles to my pool in a massive snowstorm when Gene's pool was closed. The younger team's coach indicated that he was still going to hold the practice. He lived much closer than we did and when we reached the pool, we learned that he decided not to come. It was not a happy moment since it was a heavy snowstorm and a dangerous road back and forth. Some swimmers living close to the pool showed up for practice so it was important that we persevered. It was another example of our conscience and not wanting to be seen as taking the easy way out.

The swimmers that we coached progressed very well, but the board eventually felt that they could only afford one coach at meets. The board decided that the coach who had the younger swimmers would be the coach on the deck in alternate meets. Gene did not agree with the board's decision because he wanted to be with his swimmers at all meets. He considered covering the additional expense personally for us to attend local meets, but he still was not sure that this was fair to us or the team. He then asked a crucial question, which decided our future with the team. He asked for that edict to not apply to national meets which would be held in other parts of the country. It seemed rational that the board would agree to that because it was Gene's swimmers that would most likely qualify nationally. They said that the new edict would apply. That was it. We were out of there. We would not neglect the swimmers that Gene trained by not being in charge at all their meets, especially at a national championship.

We then took coaching jobs with a relatively high-powered team in Massachusetts. Gene had that as a standing offer for a while and now decided to take it. Gene did not have to drive me to one pool and then drive to his pool miles apart. He would be the head coach for the southern portion of the team and I was the assistant coach who trained the younger swimmers. He often told people that he loved me in that position since he did not have to worry that the swimmers who moved to his group were void of the basics of competitive swimming. He also knew that they had discipline in their practice efforts. I also had no compunction to advancing swimmers, as some others might, when I thought they were ready.

We arrived on the scene, shortly after Gene had seriously injured his ankle, and was using a cane. You can imagine what was going on in the minds of the swimmers after having two much younger coaches prior to us. Were they thinking, "Were we that bad off in getting replacement coaches, that we had to settle with two old people, including one who could not get around without a cane? Were they brought out of a retirement home?"

That thinking soon vanished when the team improved so much that parents and swimmers on the northern team with more elite swimmers saw the southern team's improvement. Our section of the team, which was originally the poor stepsister, was beginning to be the envy of some of the parents on the northern team. Gene was respected by the older swimmers from the northern section and I

Gene Damm

was respected by the parents of the younger swimmers from the other section. No disrespect to their elite northern coach who owned the team and was a former Olympic coach. It was Gene's way of teaching strokes and motivating swimmers that led them to him. The older swimmers often consulted Gene prior to their races at meets. Both of us were respected by the coach owner as well.

One day when Gene was presiding over the northern section practice, he was watching a swimmer who had taken fifth in the 1500-meter freestyle at the Olympics. Gene was amazed that his turns looked so poorly executed and commented along with an estimate of what his Olympic time would have been if he had fixed them. It turns out that he might have been standing on the third-place platform rather than just being in the finals. That swimmer went on to correct his turns and won Senior Nationals, one of the top meets in a non-Olympic year. When queried by Swimming World magazine about how he felt winning at age of 28, unusual at the time for a male swimmer, he said no one should win the meet at 28. The reason that he did, Gene used to tell swimmers at our camps, was that he fixed his turns and had a will to win. Gene could never figure out why his other coaches before did not work to correct his turns. I guess it was because he was a fast swimmer and they chose not to change anything.

Lawrence became a good friend of ours after working with Gene. When Gene was paid for giving lessons at the college where we eventually coached and trained, Lawrence pointed out that his charges were too low. Just another case where Gene was charging what he thought was reasonable financially, instead of the value he provided. One of his lesson swimmer's parents said the same thing, but he kept his rates low. We are friends to this day with some of those lesson parents.

Gene had worked with two boys, the faster on his technique and the slower on both his technique and confidence. The two of them ended up as quality college swimmers. When the boys were living in

England, the older boy and one of his English swimming friends were in the United States for a camp in Florida. We flew down to watch Them. The night before the last day of the meet, the lesson swimmer's father had relayed that the English boy had not done as well as he would have liked to date and did not want to compete in the 500-meter swim the next day. The father said that he was not expecting a good race from him. Gene's answer was, "Don't bet on it." The next day the English swimmer had a great time and the lesson swimmer's father said to Gene, "How did you know that?" Gene in essence told him that it was simple. The swimmer was going out in his comfort zone and didn't want to destroy his form by exceeding his ability to control his technique. When he saw how much he was ahead, the rest was easy.

One of our lesson swimmers was a 22-time Division III All American. Gene had given her a lesson during the college break and afterwards, her coach called Gene her "stroke doctor" because she looked so much better than the other swimmers. We were invited to her wedding and are still friends.

I was a strict disciplinarian, but I also let my younger swimmers know I cared for them. Occasionally, on a Friday, I would let the swimmers get out of practice early if one of them volunteered to do a long-distance swim, usually reserved for older swimmers. Imagine the joy for both them and me in seeing a ten-year-old swimming a 400- yard individual medley or a 500-yard event while my swimmers lined up on the poolside cheering their hero on. My swimmers were not going to be afraid of these distances and I did this by showing them that it could be done by the hale and hardy. We paid attention to every swimmer on our team. That amazed one of the parents of the lesser swimmers in our section, who in the past did not get that much attention at meets. Gene's approach was that we coach everyone. We developed many lasting friends there. The team was becoming a family, almost like we had with the Saint Mary's Whalemen, our CYO team, as well as other teams we coached. The team was exceeding expectations and the wall of happiness stayed solid.

In the meantime, I decided that I should not be the only one in our immediate family without a Bachelor's degree. I decided I was going to go to college in my 50s.. During the community college part of my learning, my accomplishments were recognized with a Most Outstanding Student plaque. I went on to finish my Bachelor's degree through the Empire State College out of New York State. It involved remote learning and fit the bill for whatever location we were coaching at the time. One of the professors I chose happened to be a friend of ours. We had coached her children as competitive swimmers. She told me that she would agree to me taking her class, but be forewarned that I would receive no leeway in grading. I responded, in essence, that I would want it no other way. Getting my degree was a source of great satisfaction to me. It satisfied my intellect, and I had fun. Since I was an English/History major, it allowed me to not just satisfy my ambition, but it helped me communicate intelligently on several subjects in history.

In The Eyes of an Alzheimer's Patient

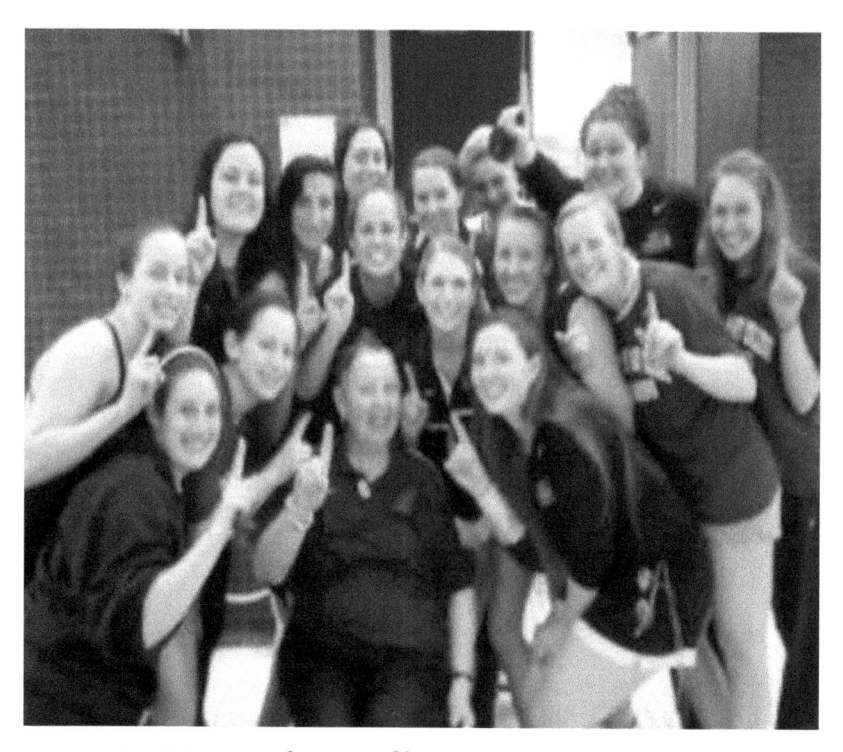

Mary with one of her winning teams

In The Eyes of an Alzheimer's Patient

Starting a New Swimming Program

In a matter of time, Gene had his second heart attack. Again, after two stents, he came back strong. He avoided a third stent, which the doctors were going to put in later as he had been on the table too long for the first two. Gene exercised by walking up and down the hills of Albuquerque, New Mexico while we were visiting our middle daughter, Erin, and her husband, Jim, at the time of the attack. The third stint was avoided thanks to this exercise regimen.

Here we go again. I decided after we resumed a similar hectic pace with a long commute to the pools where we coached, that we should move back to New York for both his health and my mental state. I missed not being close to at least part of our family. Although we were living close to our hometown of New Bedford, our schedule did not allow us to see our friends as much as we would have liked. I need not say, that I got my way. My daughter needed some parttime help in her job and Mount Saint Mary College in Newburgh, New York was starting up a swimming program which needed two coaches. This was perfect timing. The pay was almost nothing, especially for a coach of Gene's ranking, but it kept the wall of happiness intact. The important thing was our happiness.

The coach owner of the teams in New England did not want us to leave. I told him that we did not want to stay and give him a 50%

effort. His reaction was that 50% of us were more than he could get from someone else. Our decision held. We closed up the cottage and sold it to avoid more mortgage payments. We also sold the powerboat and were on our way back to New York. After we left, we found out that one of the parents, presumably in the Northern section, had anonymously donated a scholarship in our name. It was so nice of them.

Several swimmers traveled from the east coast of Massachusetts all the way to New York State to take lessons from Gene. Around that time, someone called to see if he would be interested in coaching in North Carolina. We turned that one down, guess why? We also had a call from a mother of a younger swimmer on a section of the team which we did not directly coach, except at team practices on Saturdays and at swim meets. She wanted us to come back to Massachusetts and start up a team of our own. They offered up their Cape Cod home to be our base. No rent was mentioned. Her daughter was a swimmer on the northern team, but she admired our approach to coaching and the results. It was a gracious offer, but we turned it down. It was becoming a habit. She then sent her daughter, along with the son of a very good friend, who we had coached in Massachusetts, to take a week's worth of lessons from Gene. We put them up at our house and used the college pool for lessons. There was no charge of course. These were friends, and they were still our swimmers. The boy was originally my swimmer, who did quite well but was reluctant to move up to Gene's section even though I felt that as a ten-year-old he should. He was finally convinced and eventually gained a top sixteen in the nation ranking in his age group. I felt justified in moving him up.

The team also brought us back to direct swim camps for a couple of summers. They paid us each a handsome salary and gave us room and board. They offered to put us up in a motel, but we said that we wanted to stay in the dormitory with the swimmers. The dormitory room they put us in was huge and had all the comforts of home. We were very happy with it and were close to the swimmers if they needed us. We ran the camp with coaching during the day and guest instructors in physical education and an orthopedic doctor at night. We wanted to get them well educated as well as not give them too much free time to get into trouble.

At the college in Newburgh, New York, we started up the college teams with many swimmers which had little or no experience. Gene was the coach of the men's team and I was the women's coach. As usual, we ignored the protocol as time went on. Gene handled the more experienced swimmers and I taught the others how to become competitive swimmers. We each, in this case, prepared our own line-ups for meets. With the structure of the school, I was able to attract more females, and the team grew to be a powerhouse in our conference. Our women's team won the conference, and I won coach of the year more than once thanks to our numbers and strength. My novice swimmers were not novices anymore. Gene always said that if a weaker swimmer were able to get the last scoring position by beating out an opponent, they might be the reason that our teams won meets. They would score that point and the other team would lose it. It was a double gain. The weaker swimmers reacted well to this and it helped make them more competitive. Our combined effort was another example of the team of Gene and Mary making both teams better.

I was a strict disciplinarian, and during the early morning practices, if someone did not show up, I would call the guard station and have them knock on the missing swimmer's door to wake them up for practice. I also called a commuter student's house to have his mother wake him up and have him get to practice. When some of the girls complained about all they had to do, I drew up an average day's schedule, showing them that they had plenty of time if they organized their day properly. If they came to me saying that they would have to miss practice to finish a required paper, I would ask them about when the paper was assigned to them. They knew where I was coming from. It was tough love, but they learned a lot about responsibilities.

Gene Damm

Gene, on the other hand, had a different approach. What's new? If he seemed angry, he was usually only role-playing and they knew it. He maintained discipline more by motivation than anger. One swimmer told Gene that he did not mind when Gene talked loudly to him. He really worried when Gene talked quietly.

Attracting male swimmers to the school remained a challenge, but those that did attend developed as a force of their own, even against teams with many more swimmers. At one point, Gene's team went 11-1 in dual meet competition. The only loss was against a college in Massachusetts, when his best swimmer was visiting his sick grandfather in another country. Overall, it was a very successful season. The men's team beat the traditional conference winner in their dual meet competition. That team was much larger, but our men's team was close to a peak and well-motivated. Gene was coach of the year at the end of the season. During the season, his small team had beaten the team which had gone undefeated in dual meets in the conference for a number of years. It was a close meet, ultimately decided by the last few events. It was so close that one of their swimmers decided to miss one of his classes, much to the dismay of his coach. It was the breaststroke event that would decide the meet. However, our freshman swimmer outdid himself and took the win for us. Talk about emotion from a small group of guys. Both of us were able to be undefeated in conference dual meets.

One day a male college swimmer came to me with a personal problem and asked me to listen and help him. I told him that he should know that I might not agree with him. He countered with the fact that he knew that, but I would at least be fair. What a tribute. Of course, I listened and thought that I gave him good advice.

One of the boys I really liked is now a respected oncologist. Sorry to all the boys who I told were my favorite. It was a standing joke with them. We loved our swimmers and treated them all fairly. But PJ was one of my favorites, probably because he liked to tease people in a way that did not make them angry. That part of him was just like me. He helped Gene in the early years to form a more powerful team. When the men's team did not do well at one dual meet, Gene met with the team in a conference room to discuss the surprisingly poor performance. When we arrived back at the college, PJ suggested that maybe they should consider a new beginning and solidify it by starting practices at the opposite end of the pool. Gene never stopped swimmers from giving good advice and that was implemented in the practice. Whatever magic was taking place, the men finished the season with great performances. Gene used the word "focus" in the college practices so much that PJ gave him a stone paperweight with the word "focus" engraved in it. Thanks, PJ.

When PJ was first interning in pediatric oncology, I said to Gene, "Poor PJ", thinking that he would be saddened by the cases he dealt with. Gene's reaction was, "Are you kidding? He is a little imp," (which he was) "and the kids will love him." I lost track of the fact that making the children happy would mollify his own sadness. A copy of his graduation picture with us was placed in my casket as a remembrance.

One of the fun memories with the college team was when we were on a training trip in Orlando, Florida. At Disney Springs, there was a circular area in the walkway that would suddenly spurt out streams of water. I danced in the area with one of my swimmers as the water shot up on us. We had great fun. Too bad Gene could not find the video to show you.

Gene Damm

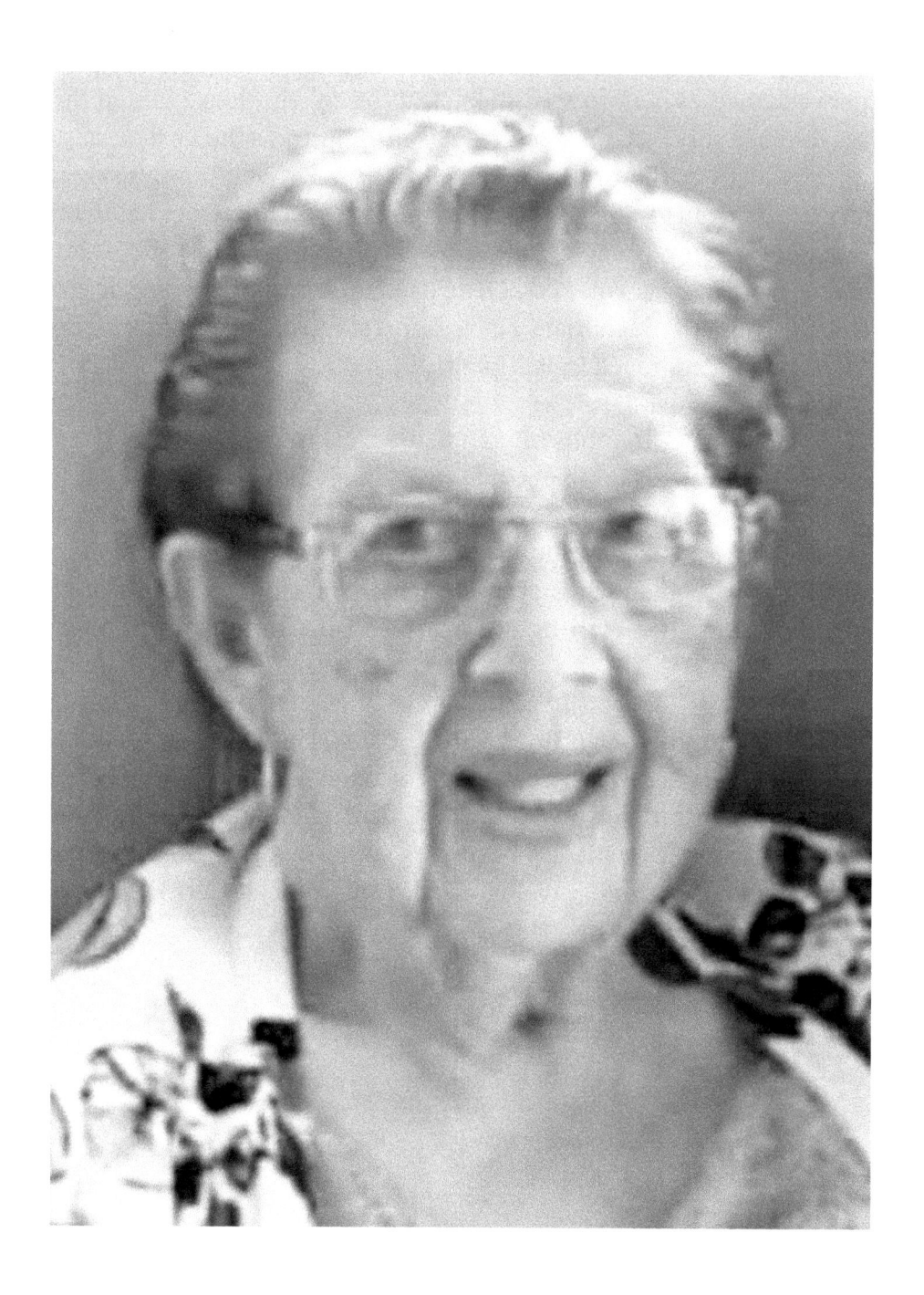

A Bump in the Road

During our time at Mount Saint Mary College, I was diagnosed with both diabetes and breast cancer. Gene had sensed something was wrong, even though I tried to hide the breast cancer. He talked to our daughters about it. Two of my daughters, one of them from across the country, a nurse, and our oldest daughter came to our house. They sent Gene out of the room, so he would not be tempted to give in to me. My daughters said, "You are going to get checked out." Our youngest daughter would have come, but she had her own problems with a sick husband. Gene had the sense to call them when I was obstinate about my health. I immediately was sent to the hospital where I had a mastectomy.

Fortunately, they were able to remove all of the cancer, and with the post-op treatments, there was no recurrence. All through the radiation and chemotherapy, I continued to coach. Only once did Gene direct me to go into the pool office during a meet when I was exhausted from the chemotherapy. At one of the meets, a priest who knew that I was receiving chemotherapy, said that I was a tough old bird. I did not mind the words tough or bird, but I resented being told that I was old and the connotations that go with that. I was still sharp as could be, not knowing that I would ever change. At that point, it was getting tough, but I was tougher. Little did I know the horrible nature of the disease that was about to overtake me.

When Gene was diagnosed with prostate cancer, in his early 70s, he wanted a second opinion on treatment at his age and chose a group at Massachusetts General Hospital. They were highly respected in their field for this type of second opinion. The group even included a psychiatrist. We traveled there and the group of doctors suggested that he have radiation with hormone treatments rather than surgery. His local heart doctor said that he could survive the surgery if he chose that instead, but he chose radiation. This was mainly because he did not want to be out of the college practice that long, even though it was riskier for his long-term survival at the time. How is that for smarts? We continued to coach after those events. That was our passion and nothing was going to stop us, or so we thought.

During the strong hormone treatments prior to radiation, he suffered hot flashes in the warm indoor pool area but kept going. None of the swimmers would ever know that he had prostate cancer unless they read this book. It turned out that the procedure was so successful that his urologist, who had previously not liked radiation as a solution, told him that he might now choose it for himself if he ever had prostate cancer. Will wonders never cease. He survived what could have been a life-threatening decision, and changed a doctor's bias.

When the college needed a new aquatic director, they appointed Gene to that job in addition to his coaching responsibilities. It also was not much pay, but he was the person that the athletic director trusted when it came to the pool. I of course ended up, by my choice, helping him with the process of scheduling lifeguards and doing the resulting paperwork that went with it. Ours was always a team effort.

In his added role, Gene had a number of issues with the athletic director, even though they were friends. The athletic director was mainly worried about budget and recruiting. He let Gene take care of the pool, but it was different when it came to finances. Gene's idea of a budget is that it should be lean, but there should be a contingency factor at some level to take care of the inevitable and unexpected emergencies. You plan for the expected, and while keeping the budget realistically lean, be protected for the unexpected.

Any contingency money could then not be touched without upper management approval. Gene's point also was that all rules, no matter how strict, must be ready to have a waiver if there is a valid reason for it. Such a case arose when the round plastic rings on the divider lane rope started leaving chips of plastic in the pool. Gene's request to replace them was turned down for budget reasons. Gene confronted the athletic director and told him that a high school team renting the pool brought in thousands of dollars and he would not put in bad lane lines, nor would he accept responsibility for the liability if one of the swimmers swallowed a sharp plastic chip. No lane ropes, no income from meets, no home meets for the college team, and perhaps restricted practices for both teams to accommodate the numbers without divider ropes. We suddenly got new lane ropes.

There were other conflicts on liability and budget. One of them came with a recreational camp director who was also the principal of the elementary school on the college campus. There were issues about how many lifeguards and counselors should be in the pool observing the 10 and under campers. Gene was strict on this, especially when he heard that in one pool, a very young boy drowned when the teacher lost sight of him while he was watching the other five under his guidance. They did not like Gene's rules, but he was in control. His pool safety rules would also have been reinforced by the local Board of Health. A government rule was enacted for spas and pools, but for some reason, it did not come under the local Board of Health to enforce. Gene convinced his athletic director that the liability was still there. Gene also heard that during a meeting of the Board of Health, the manager said that she was sure that Gene would be one of the people who would enforce it at the college pool.

Gene Damm

One major issue with the elementary school camp got escalated to our athletic director. The power source for controlling humidity failed and the pool area became very uncomfortable. The camp director wanted to leave an exit door open to alleviate the problem. Gene said that he would open it only if one of the counselors or adults had an EpiPen and could administer it should a bee, or wasp, fly in and sting an allergic swimmer. Gene thought that the precaution was a no-brainer. We were at a grocery store having a bagel and coffee when the call came in. The athletic director was extremely upset, to say the least. He said then that he wanted Gene to open the door. The school principal, who was sitting there listening, had complained to him. Gene explained his position, but could not get many words in while the athletic director was chewing him out. This was not going well in my mind, because I knew Gene did not appreciate being chewed out when he was right. Instead of breaking in with an angry voice, he said something I would never have said to my boss. Addressing him by his first name, he said 'Take three breaths and listen to me. Maintenance is building a special screen door which should be ready later today or tomorrow. Once the screen door is installed, I will open the door when the pool is in use. It would be a comfort to the lifeguards as well as the campers." The conversation ended, maybe not as graciously as it could have been, but it ended.

Gene also had a fixation on the fact that when there is a problem, you do not shoot the messenger. We were on vacation one day and Gene found out that a different member of the Board of Health had been in the pool area. The lifeguard could not find the copy of our safety plan, so she rummaged through Gene's desk and found a prior one. The Board of Health member chastised the lifeguard as she apparently did to the staff at the restaurants that she normally visited. Gene did not like that approach. He called the manager of the Board of Health and stated that the new safety plan was under a pile on the table at poolside at the time of the visit and that they also had a copy of it in their office which he had sent them when it was created. He ended up telling them that if they had a problem, they should take it up with him, not the lifeguard. The manager agreed and had a meeting with her whole staff to advise them of the proper procedure. Their normal staff member from there was strict on rules, but very friendly and helped Gene with data on pool procedures. Gene remains friendly with that person, even after both have retired.

In another situation, a visiting high school team coach harassed one of the lifeguards when she approached him to discuss something. Gene did not like his lifeguards being harassed unfairly. When he heard about the situation, he ended up calling their athletic director and told him that if this continued, they would not be able to compete in a meet with the local teams at our pool. At their next meet, the coach denied that he was harassing the lifeguard and Gene repeated what the coach had apparently said. The coach behaved well after that. That was my Gene, a man of complexity. He was normally pleasant and even submissive to good ideas but was unbelievably strong when he had to be. I do not like to boast, but will let you know that I helped him master this demeanor. The one thing I did not change, nor did I want to, was his passion for competitiveness. As quiet and as gracious as he was, when he or our teams were not at the top, he worked hard to change that. He certainly was not a quitter and always felt that things could improve if you worked hard enough from both the coach and the swimmer aspect. He was more competitive than many people realized from his calm composure.

Gene Damm

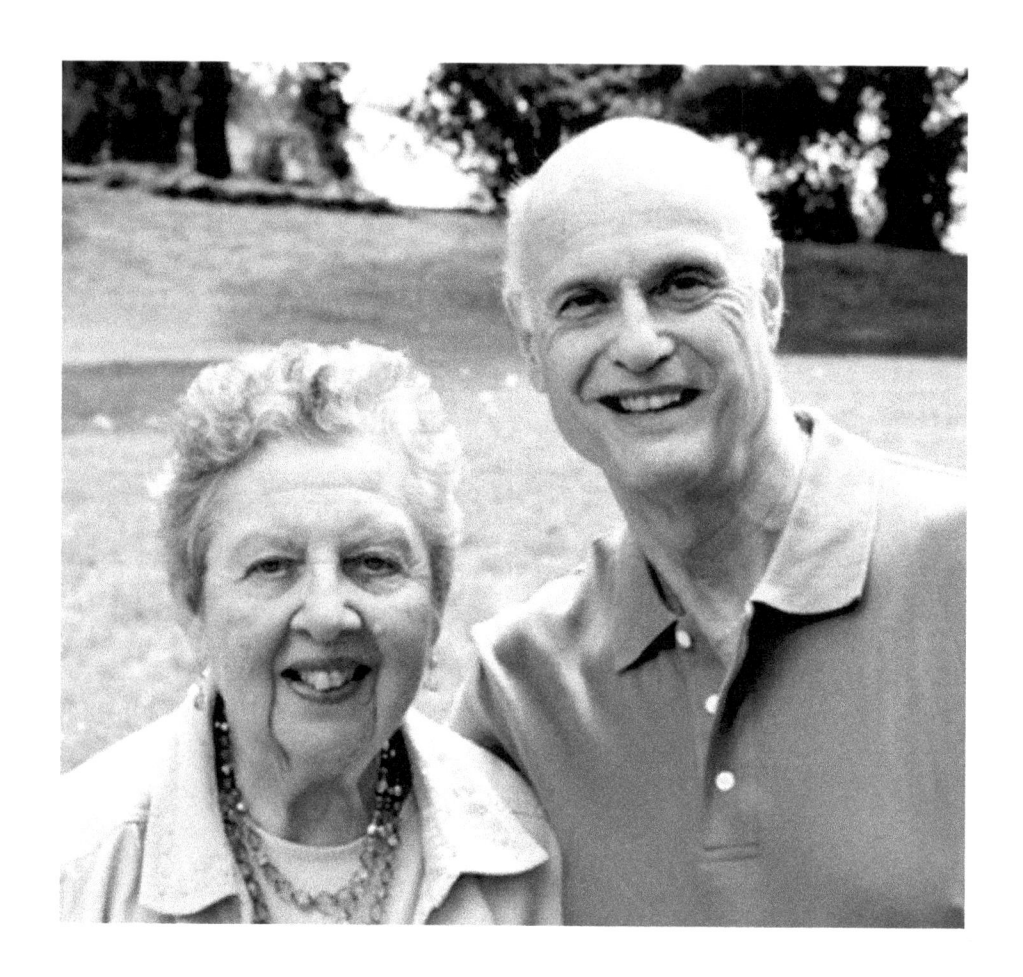

A Major Bump in the Road

Gene was in his late 70s when another large bump in the road occurred. Gene tripped on an upturned area rug and hit his head hard on the corner of the door frame. He had a concussion. Shortly after that he had a kidney stone and was given a medicine to relieve it. Unbeknown to him, the medicine was originally developed as a hypertensive drug, and when he took it at night with his blood pressure medicine, he fainted. His condition worsened, but he thought that the original concussion might not have healed yet, and did not want to go back to the doctor and sound foolish.

Eventually, Gene's condition deteriorated to such an extent that our oldest daughter drove him to a neurologist who sent him to the hospital immediately for further evaluation. By the time he got there, he was out of it and thought our oldest son-in-law was one of our daughters. That was not the father that our oldest daughter knew. She insisted that it was not old age creeping up on him as the emergency room staff was trying to convince us that it was. Our family doctor, when called in, reinforced our belief and said that Gene should be tested. He knew Gene well. With the doctor on our side, the hospital then proceeded to order tests, including a CT scan on his head.

The CT scan showed a very large bleed and a neurosurgeon was called in. He told us that we only had a couple of minutes to decide on whether to have surgery to address the problem. We were also warned that there was only a 50-50 chance of success. The family held a conference by phone and we all agreed to the operation, praying for success. I was a nervous wreck. It was really me following their lead. An operating room nurse visited Gene a day or two later to see how he was doing and told him that when they bored the first hole through his skull the blood shot across the operating room. Gene was glad that he was not that doctor since he would have kneejerked and spoiled the operation. He spent a long time in recovery and rehabilitation to regain the use of his right leg, but all in all, he was a very lucky man. Thanks to many prayers and the skill of the surgeon.

Just think of what would have happened to someone who was of an advanced age and possibly even suffering from early dementia, if the family heeded the first impression of that medical professional. It is tragic that even people in the medical field can think that any change in mental acuity is attributable to old age.

Gene still planned to go back to college coaching, but abandoned that plan after our oldest daughter asked him if he really wanted to continue at his age to get home at 10:00 p.m. from the late practices every weeknight during the college season? He was 78 at the time. He may have yielded because he was still recovering from the brain bleed, but he did agree to retirement and liked to always keep his word. We retired from college coaching. Even though we spent a lot of time at the pool, both as aquatic directors and coaches, we were considered parttime employees and there was no pension. After we left Mount Saint Mary, they hired a full-time coach and aquatic director at a higher cost. It was inevitable if they wanted to find a qualified person to equal our joint efforts. The first coach they hired had quit the first day because they had added too much to the job to justify the salary.

In The Eyes of an Alzheimer's Patient

With that phase of our life behind us, and Gene still recovering, I convinced him to volunteer to help a former swimmer now coaching a local swim team. It ended up being a three-day-a-week job. This helped keep Gene's passion for coaching alive. He was still in recovery so he had to be careful on a wet deck, but he survived that. The parents and swimmers appreciated his assistance with their stroke technique. During those three days, practices were 4:00 p.m. to 6:00 p.m, so we ended up most nights with a sandwich at the pool for dinner. We were usually very early, but if we were delayed for some reason, Gene had his sandwich while he was on the deck as a coach. That was a throwback to when we used to eat in the car while traveling to various activities. I, in turn, would eat while waiting for him and talking to the parents.

Gene worked with a former swimmer of his who coached the senior swimmers and they got along fabulously. Most of the time, I would be chatting with the wonderful mothers. We often laughed together. It was one of my favorite times. We loved all of the people and swimmers that we met on the team. We even sometimes went to lunch with several of the parents. We also met for ice cream with two of the mothers that we were especially friendly. Gene and I were addicted to ice cream, especially homemade ice cream. So, between the ice cream and the company, we had a great time. It was in the selection of the flavor of ice cream that we were also dramatically different. I loved chocolate and Gene did not like chocolate. He loved butter pecan but would select other flavors when it was not available. Chocolate was not usually an option. It took a while to reach common "ground." It was another of our Jack Spratt and his wife analogies. When we found a place near a pool with homemade ice cream, we would occasionally stop there.

We did both like coffee ice cream, which was a product of our Massachusetts upbringing. Coffee ice cream was one of our favorites since our families would even buy coffee syrup to add to our milk to help us enjoy our milk more. I loved Dunkin' Donuts coffee and we usually stopped for coffee on the way to the pool just about every day and again at night if we were coming back from a meet. I would get iced coffee, even in the middle of winter, and Gene would get hot coffee even in the middle of summer. It was still another difference in our likes and dislikes. He usually went in for the coffees. At times he bought me a DD baseball cap, a DD stocking cap, and a lunch pail to demonstrate my love for coffee. The man, who did not do much for himself, bought these things for me. I deserved them. He might say that it was for putting up with him.

Gene was comfortable with the mothers who were at the pool. After all, he was brought up before his family separated, with two sisters, and he had a wife, three daughters, and a female dog. He did joke that even the voice on our GPS was another female voice telling him what to do. He used another quip at the pool stating that it was twenty years after our marriage that he finally learned that his nickname was not "Stupid." I had taught him well to joke, but now he was incorrigible.

He was also friendly with the fathers that came to the pool and became very good friends with one who also had a scientific background. Gene chats with him even now. They had some interesting discussions which I could not totally understand, but I knew that they enjoyed talking together. This gentleman and his wife, along with a widow friend I was friendly with, later made a point of visiting us at our home in Florida. This bond was secure, and Gene and several of the parents from the team still correspond by phone. We also have day visits and calls from parents of lesson swimmers that we befriended when they were vacationing in Florida.

Eventually, Gene helped another team as well, which made four nights of volunteering. The coach really appreciated his stroke technique work. He also would have liked me to coach because he had a friend from Rhode Island whom I had coached and they spoke very highly of me. I was not able to help on the pool deck because my illness was at a stage that I could not. However, it was a beautiful compliment to the second half of the team of Gene and Mary. After we moved to Florida, the coach initiated a special award for his swimmers and named it the Gene and Mary Damm Perseverance award as a tribute to us. It is a special honor which we did not expect, but it was, and is, greatly appreciated. My sharing the honor with Gene proved that good swimmers were developed by our teamwork. Gene often still talks with those coaches.

A couple of years or so after we retired, we were both elected to the Hall of Fame at Mount Saint Mary College. Our prior Hall of Fame recognition had been by the Duchess County Sports Museum for our work with young swimmers. At the college Hall of Fame night, we chose the senior age group coach Gene was volunteering for, who was one of our former swimmers, to introduce us. He cited our accomplishments, noting what an important role we played in his life. Gene had me go first to talk as he usually did. The coach who introduced us was worried about my memory and later said to Gene that he was surprised at how eloquent my speech was. I guess my memory or lack thereof was beginning to be noticeable, but I hadn't really thought too much about it yet. Alzheimer's was just starting to show its ugly head.

When Gene got up to talk, he, as usual, said that my talk covered everything that he would have said. He then proceeded to give a talk about a major sports person who said that the reason he had won with a record time under adverse, supposedly life-threatening conditions, was that he had to get over a mental block and had to have the will to do it. He then proceeded essentially to say that it was easy to coach, but the swimmer had to have the determination to execute what the coach was trying to say. The athlete deserves much credit for believing in their coach.

The following picture of the Hall of Fame night shows two young ladies who were lifeguards for us. They are still friends with us and they visit us in Florida. One time, the two of them stayed with us in our mobile home for a few days. We had a great time, and to show us their appreciation, they took us to an opera in Sarasota. It was my first opera and the show was fantastic.

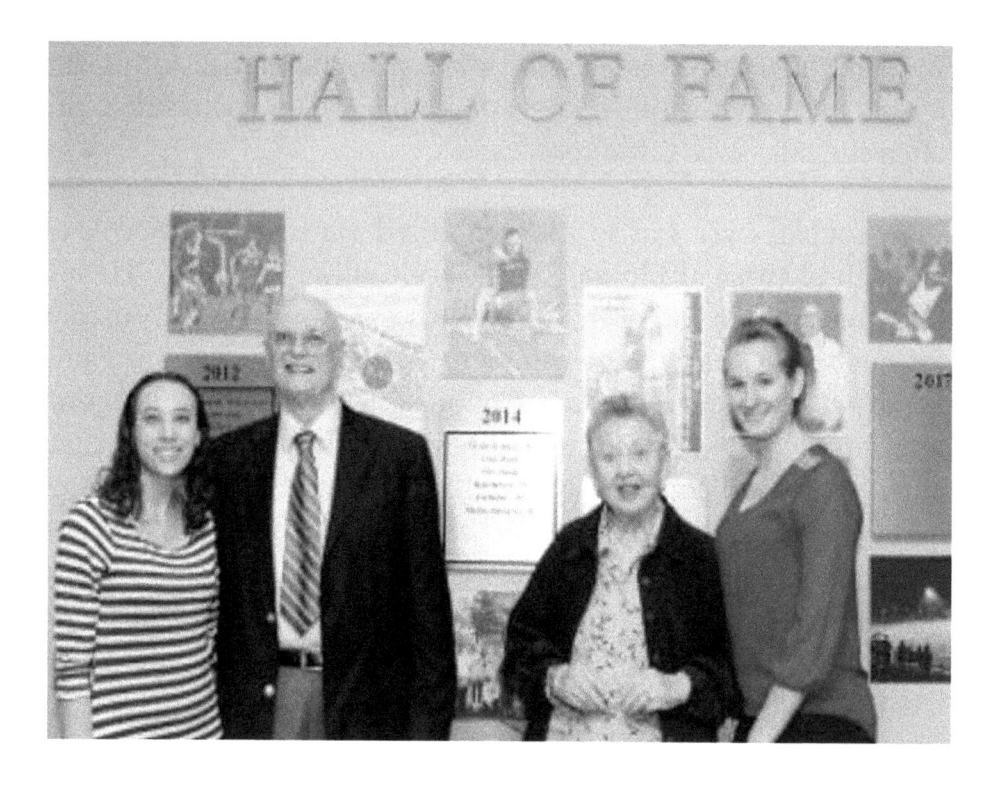

Two of our Former Lifeguards (Friends to this day)

The wall of happiness was still strong, albeit probably a little strenuous for us. We were still tough. The only glitch was that my illness was beginning to show up.

I loved to shop, and once a week we would take our oldest daughter's mother-in-law out with us and have lunch. Her husband had passed and we were all pretty close. She even vacationed with us at our timeshare on Cape Cod. I loved Cape Cod and its proximity to New Bedford. Not to mention the good seafood and Portuguese food. I also loved their homemade ice cream which was part of our daily routine.

I would buy clothes on sale, although many I never wore. I especially enjoyed buying things for our great-grandchildren. I loved our family and would even buy clothes for the little ones to start school. I sent checks out for Halloween and Valentine's Day, which I jokingly called Naked Baby Angel Day. If I bought something for Gene, he would kid me by saying that I had a guilt complex because he hardly ever bought anything for himself. You can make your own decision as to whether there was any truth to that.

Our oldest granddaughter, Kimberly, mentioned that she had told her daughter how at Christmas time, Gene would walk out to the car in her parent's driveway several times to bring in big green garbage bags filled with wrapped gifts I had bought. I loved my children, grandchildren, and great-grandchildren, and aside from the religious aspect of Christmas, it was a special time to show that love. I know, you will say that I spoiled them, but doesn't that happen to lots of people with their grandchildren and great-grandchildren? One year, one of our grandsons said that I was not to buy more than three things for Christmas for his girls. My retort was that stocking suffers and clothes do not count. I was incorrigible, even when it came to non-clothing. In the end, they got lots of clothes and more toys. I think that underneath, my grandson knew that he was asking the impossible.

If we were on a trip and I had brought clothes that I had not worn before, Gene would ask if they were new? When I said that I had worn them before, he said, "How come the tag is still on it?" His favorite tease with the college swimmers was, "She was never like this when she babysat me." So much for me teaching him how to wisecrack. My retort was that I would never have babysat a brat like him. Speaking of spending, I always told him that he should treat himself with a luxury car, but to him, his current car was good enough, cheaper to repair, and had good mileage. Try to fight that, even though I kept saying that right to the end of my communicative life.

Gene Damm

I saw the local great-grandchildren often and used to recite the mouse went up the clock story for them as I ran my fingers up their arm. I earned the name of "Mousey" from them, and that is what they always called me. I even received a hat that had Mousey embroidered on it. The name certainly did not fit the dictionary definition of the word "mousy," or "mousey," whichever you prefer. But in their minds, it fit me as the mouse storyteller. After my passing, they mourned me more than I would have believed, including wearing my jewelry that Gene had given them as a tribute. I had teased one of them with nicknames, and months after my passing, at eight years old, she would cry, reliving how she missed me and my teasing. The times visiting our other great-grandchildren in Oregon were also a treasure, but unfortunately, we were not able to see them that much.

We had a great family life. On Sundays, Tom and Mary would drive us to church along with his mother. After church, we would all have breakfast together at a local diner. There was usually enough food for us to take our leftovers to the senior center where we met our middle daughter's mother and father-in-law on Mondays. My middle daughter's father-in-law liked to say controversial things and I would disagree with him. Gene used to say he did that deliberately to get a response out of me. He sure got one. We were friends with them, as we were with our youngest son-in-law's widowed mother. And of course, our oldest daughter's mother-in-law. We did not see as much of our youngest daughter's widowed mother-in-law who lived in Connecticut, but we were able to have some good conversations over the phone, also producing a special relationship. Our family and extended family were all wonderful to us. All three daughters had given us not only sons, grandchildren, and great-grandchildren, but also many new friends.

We had swimmers of all ages that were like sons and daughters to us. The college swimmers had described us as a grandmother and grandfather to them. Many of our former swimmers of all ages cared enough to still talk to Gene online and through social media. I did not understand, nor did I want to understand computers and texting, so the correspondence was carried on by Gene. He usually kept me up to date and it was great that a number of our swimmers and college lifeguards remained in contact with us.

Many of our swimmers have entered professions that help others. Some in the medical professions of doctoring and nursing, as well as teaching, firefighting, and police work, along with coaching to a great success I might add. We are more than proud of them, since helping and servicing others was one of the professions that we chose. We are also proud of our past swimmers in other professions I have not mentioned.

Gene Damm

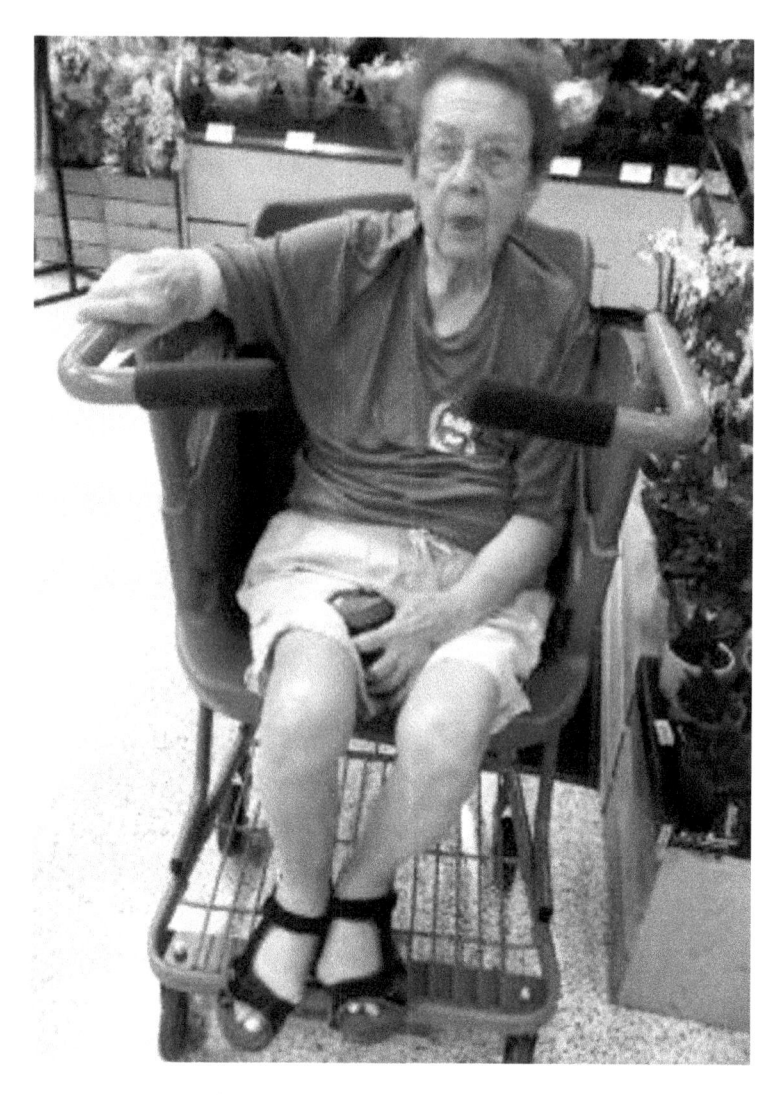

Mary out shopping thanks to Publix at Skywalk

In The Eyes of an Alzheimer's Patient

The Wall Starts to Crumble

I did not know when my Alzheimer's started. I may have progressed from a person of reasonably higher intelligence to one of average intelligence to a person whose inability to remember was due to some kind of early dementia. But let the story of that begin.

Around 2015, among the usual failures in memory, there was also a change in my personality, I became more irritated at times, and at other times submissive to medical tests that I would ordinarily reject.

There was another change, though; a warning sign that something was wrong with me. I was always a very precise person who followed my bookkeeping background explicitly. We had a small checking account for money earned from Gene's lessons, that we used to pay associated bills and keep them separate from our regular account. I started randomly writing checks on that account for other items that exceeded the balance. Fortunately, my daughter Mary was joint on the account, and she fixed things. When she looked at our bank statements, she found a number of them unopened. That was not me. Also, when I wrote checks, instead of removing them neatly, I would just rip them out with all jagged pieces on the top. If my grandchildren received a check in an envelope, they knew who it was from without looking at the signature, It made for fun, but it was a wide deviation from the normal me. While these changes were almost unnoticeable it was the start of the new me and my new personality. The early stages of Alzheimer's may be difficult to detect but watch for other little changes, as well as the usual memory loss.

I was in my 80's when somehow my legs did not want to respond as well as they use to. My short-term memory was getting shorter, but doesn't almost everyone's get shorter as they age? The first recognition that something might be seriously wrong was when we were visiting with our middle daughter, Erin, her husband, Jim, and their family in Oregon. The bedrooms were a short flight upstairs, but with help, I was able to navigate them. I was also having some serious incontinence problems, along with memory issues, all attributed to old age.

As I came down the stairs with difficulty one morning, I needed more help than usual. At breakfast, I was acting strange and my daughter thought that I had blacked out for a short time. Off we went to the hospital where they checked me out thoroughly. I thought that they only saw what might have been a minor stroke.

When I was close to being released, they asked me a number of random questions. I did great on most of them and even could count backwards from 100. Gene thought that I was doing quite well. However, they asked me some simple questions and I gave them wrong answers. My family was then told that I should not be close to cooking stoves. They also suggested that I see a neurologist when I got back home. They must have seen something more disturbing in their tests than I realized, but did not want to draw too many conclusions without further testing.

My daughter had rented a wheelchair for me because I was having trouble walking any distance at this time. Of all things, my oldest great-grandson wanted to push me through the stores. He was so young that the shoppers marveled at him doing it.

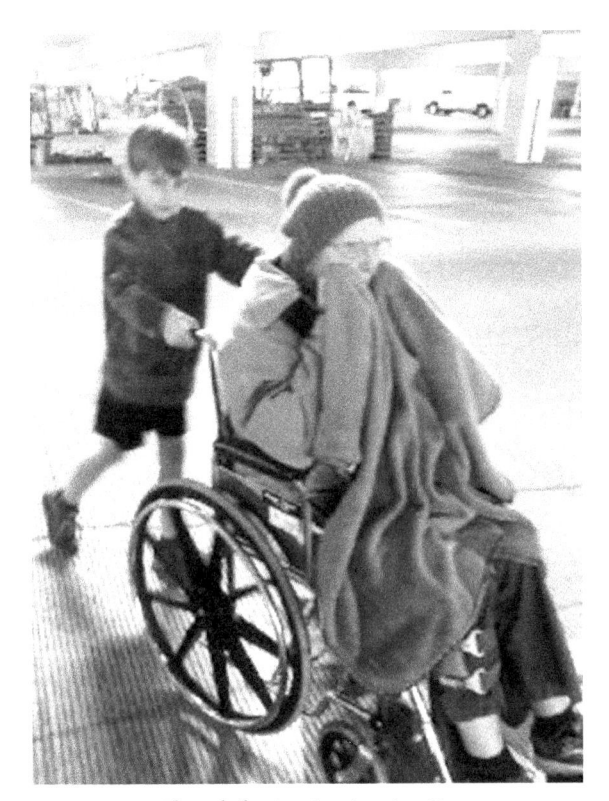

Wheelchair Assist in Oregon

During our visits to Oregon, Erin and Gene used to walk up and down several steep hills in the neighborhood, and I mean steep. Gene had walked around the hills before, but this hike was more than three miles non-stop. There had been a rest break the day before and Gene thought that he could handle it again, but this one was non-stop. That's my silly (polite word) husband. At the end of the walk, he was swinging his right leg to walk and looked like he was drunk. Erin thought that he might have had a stroke. Off to the hospital they went. After a battery of tests, they decided that the issue was a result of the problem he had after the brain bleed when he had to be taught how to use his right leg again. They dismissed him and he went back to Erin and Jim's house with no more after effects. It was interesting that the emergency room doctor in Oregon called after we got back to New York to see if Gene was still alright. What a nice doctor. I guess that he was a little bit worried about the diagnosis. But our visits to our family in Oregon left them fraught with concerns for our health.

As the enemy Alzheimer's was creeping up on me, an optometrist noticed I had acute vision loss in my left eye. He suggested that I have an ophthalmologist look at my eyes, and he in turn had me see a retinal doctor. I refused to see him as early as I should have, as you know I feared that doctors would find something seriously wrong and did not want to hear it. A short time later, I was talked into an appointment. When I went to him, it was diagnosed with wet macular degeneration, and even with very expensive shots of Eylea injected directly into the eye, they could not save it from its degradation. Although I did not end up completely blind, the vision in my left eye was as close as it could be to being blind. The Eylea did help with my right eye, but I still ended up with limited vision in that eye. Gene also noticed that I had a problem differentiating between colors.

My daughter urged me to see several doctors. I'd had my share of doctors already, so this didn't sit well with me. Urging is another polite word for tough love. Most of these visits to doctors were at the strong insistence of one or more of our daughters. Gene knew that they were more effective than him. That's because he did not have to worry about giving in to me when I rebelled. When he sensed something was seriously wrong, the "Female Reserve Corps" was called in to do the dirty work of telling me, not suggesting to me, that I should go to seek medical attention. He learned a big lesson about how ineffective he was in convincing me to see a doctor and how effective they could be.

As things got worse, my ability to walk and hold my balance was getting very troublesome. At one point when Gene was helping me get out of a car in the Walmart parking lot in Fishkill, New York, I fell and took Gene down with me when he tried to catch me. Gene was lucky that he landed on his backside rather than his head. An EMT group was coincidentally there at the time, and they helped me up to my walker. Some gentleman who saw the incident got me some water from a machine and refused Gene's offer to repay him. What a nice guy.

Our first primary doctor in Florida at the time thought I had only vascular dementia. Many times, when Alzheimer's is just beginning to show symptoms, it is diagnosed as vascular dementia. He tried to assure me that it was not critical. However, at Erin's persistence, I finally had appointments for neurological testing. The neurologist thought differently.

I ended up with neurological testing and an MRI. Earlier, I had panicked when entering the closed unit MRI machine and they were not able to complete the test. They reverted to an open MRI machine. I had extreme panic about the tests, especially with Alzheimer's leading the way, but they convinced me that an open unit would not be a problem. The conclusion was that I had both a prior stroke and a case of Alzheimer's. I was put on medicine, that they thought might cause a slight delay in my deterioration. I was told to listen to music as it would be good for me.

When the neurologist announced that I had Alzheimer's, in my typical fashion, I said, "Does that mean I am not ready for the funny farm?" It was a strange way to put it when I should have been alarmed, but it was the only joke I could think of. He must have thought that I said that I was ready for the funny farm and came back to me saying, "Don't say that, Erin will get mad at me." Our daughters always took care of us in our older years, and have no compunction to talk to the doctors if they feel they need to amplify on what we have told them. In this case, it was Erin, our nurse daughter, who was in constant contact with our doctors. She had even set up some of the appointments.

When Gene, the everlasting scientist, saw the seven stages of Alzheimer's in his research for this book, it was apparent that I had gone through all of these stages. At this time of my disease, though, I was at stage 4.

To complicate everything, at one point, I stopped making hemoglobin and was hospitalized for several days. The hospital did not immediately have a room for me and my doctor suggested that I change hospitals. The hospital nurse said that it would be difficult, since I had already been checked in. They then moved me up to a closet until a room was found. It turned out to be a good decision to keep me in that hospital since I received excellent care. The doctor's ordered two blood transfusions, along with iron infusions to kickstart the recovery of the hemoglobin in my blood. Gene stayed with me throughout the day and made sure that he got instant feedback on the results. The team finally raised my hemoglobin back to a reasonable level. It then became a bump in the road. One of many bumps that became larger and larger at this stage of my life.

There was also a time in Florida when I was further along with Alzheimer's. We were in a Target store when Gene had to make some purchases. He brought me in the store and positioned me in my walker in the front of the store rather than pushing me around while he shopped. Leaving me in the car was not an option. At that time my zeal to shop and walk around the store was a distant memory and I really did not mind sitting and waiting. The air-conditioner was set very high and I was shivering. A kind lady, who noticed me, gave me her sweater. Even though Gene was coming back shortly, without thinking, I accepted it. Gene was mortified when he saw this. The woman who had helped me had left and he did not know how to find her. We left the sweater in a conspicuous spot, near where I had been sitting, hoping that she would find it. Another perfect example of nice people in this world. Gene usually made sure that we carried a blanket or sweater in the car after that. Two of Gene's cardigans were lost in the process. I also used blankets and sweaters in the house in Florida because I was always cold, even when visitors were too warm.

In The Eyes of an Alzheimer's Patient

One embarrassing event for Gene was when I was in for one of my frequent blood tests and I lost control of my bowels. I messed myself and the room so badly that they had to close it temporarily for cleaning. Gene escorted me out the back door.

An earlier event, when we were back in Poughkeepsie, should have given me a warning about my physical health. An ultrasound that my heart doctor's office had performed showed that my heart was running with only a 30% ejection fraction, which was not good, but survivable. My doctor decided that he would order a CT scan of my heart. My family convinced me that the test was easy, and I trusted my new heart doctor, so I agreed to it, even though I had a great fear of all such tests. They did not find any blockage, so the only issue was the blood flow but, if it got worse, it would not be survivable. Would Alzheimer's take me out of this world before that happened, as it raced to destroy my mind, and thus my ability to survive? Or would it be a combination of both? Alzheimer's was not considered as serious as what was going on with my heart at the time. In Gene's mind, Alzheimer's eventually won out, as it destroyed my ability to do things to survive. As my desire to eat faded, my body did not have the necessary ingredients to carry on. It destroyed me by taking away my ability to nourish my body with the necessary ingredients to help my heart continue to beat without assistance from the rest of my body.

My Alzheimer's was beginning to be more evident. Once I got angry at a close friend at the pool where Gene was coaching. Prior to that Gene was always the target of my anger, some of it would be unfair, but he was the only safe place to vent without permanently offending innocent victims. Fortunately, this friend understood.

One of the more embarrassing examples of my early Alzheimer's was when we attended a swimmer's graduation party at their home with a number of their friends, most of whom we did not know, and they did not know us. When we were about to leave, Gene suggested that I use the bathroom. Unfortunately, the bathroom was in use and the door was locked. I was impatient and began yelling and screaming unmercifully while banging on the door for the person to get out. I probably scared him and shocked the other guests. Fortunately, the hostess had someone in her family afflicted with Alzheimer's and understood. We remained friends.

When it was time to visit Florida again, our oldest daughter, Mary, and her husband, Tom, traveled with us. They used the excuse that we should see the house they had bought in Davenport, Florida. The real reason, I believe, is that they did not want us to travel alone in my condition. On an earlier trip to Oregon, Mary and Tom had us change our flight to a non-stop flight and then drove us to Newark airport to ensure that we got on without a major problem. Mary even convinced them to let her through security to help us to the gate. They did not have the confidence that Gene would be able to handle a difficult situation at his age, so their trip to Davenport was not entirely coincidental with our going to our home in North Port for what was supposed to be a three-month stay. Gene knew that his age was a factor in their decision, and while he usually agreed with his daughters and me, Gene never liked the fact that they considered him too old to be able to handle things by himself. I will not add my usual comments to this.

The Florida trip did not go as well as we would have wished. Alzheimer's can be very punishing to a person traveling with it. When we arrived in Davenport, I was in a funk and not the musical kind, but a state of depression. It got worse from there, and I had another trip to the hospital. I was diagnosed with congestive heart failure and atrial fibrillation. Gene had a hospital stay himself. As he was walking through the hospital, he was dragging his foot through the corridor and there was some concern of a stroke. It turned out to be the symptoms he also had in Oregon. His system had again, merely reverted to the symptoms he had with the brain bleed, this time it occurred because he was overtired and stressed. Gene sometimes foolishly pushes himself too far. I did not say anything to him about this. Diplomacy can be a virtue. I wish I could have had more of it, but I don't know that I ever would have achieved it. People seemed to accept my teasing and candidness, and I was happy with that. Fortunately, this event was not serious, but Tom and Mary diplomatically forced the issue that he should be checked out, given all the stressful issues confronting him.

Alzheimer's patients sometimes have trouble with travel so a decision had to be made as to whether we were going to move to Florida, or to another house in Poughkeepsie. We had talked earlier about moving to Florida, but my hospitalization cinched it for Gene. He was not going to go back to a house whose only access was up a flight of stairs. Tom had put a second railing on the other side of the stairs, but in my condition and Gene's, it would have been a major problem to hold me if I started to fall. Jim and Erin had wanted us to be near them since Erin is a nurse and could readily take care of me. Jim had a good job at Intel and Erin's job at a health company allowed her to work remotely so we were assured that someone would be with me if Gene was not available. Thinking it over with our family, we thought that Florida was our best option. Leaving our friends and Gene leaving the swim teams where he volunteered was a tough decision, but we had to make it.

We had bought a mobile home in North Port, Florida several years before, a few doors down from a dear friend from high school. It gave us a few weeks, and eventually months of vacation. She and her husband were very helpful, and the neighbors were great. There were a number of activities that my friend from high school encouraged me to enjoy. They had dances as well as sports activities for Gene along with family dinners. Gene played shuffleboard and ping pong to keep himself busy. Staying a few months, rather than a few weeks, finalized the end of Gene's volunteer coaching up north.

The mobile home had three steps into the unit, which was a disadvantage, but manageable for me at the time we bought it. We'd previously remodeled the kitchen and bathrooms in case we ever decided to permanently move there. Unfortunately, we had replaced the main bathroom tub with a full-sized one, rather than a walk-in shower. Alzheimer's had not yet visibly shown itself, so it seemed reasonable at the time.

Our youngest daughter Kathleen and her husband George had moved to Fort Myers earlier as a result of George's need for a liver transplant. George was on disability from Webster bank where he'd managed a couple of banks, and Florida was judged as one of the states where transplants were more readily available, so they moved there. Kathleen, who was a vice-president of the Wire Room at Webster Bank accepted a lesser position at a Florida bank to be with him. Gene decided that our best choice would be to move to Fort Myers to be near them, even though the mobile home was only three-quarters of an hour away.

We needed a different housing arrangement due to my illness catching up with me, making it difficult and eventually impossible for me to bathe in a bathtub. A walk-in shower was an absolute requirement in the main bathroom, in any house we would buy. Gene did not want to move into an assisted living faculty or a duplex villa because I could get very angry, and loud. We needed to buy a one-story house in Fort Myers, nearer to Kathy and George, so we ended up selling both homes. It was going to be difficult to sell the Poughkeepsie house without us being there to make it presentable for sale along with clearing out our belongings and furniture. The burden would have to fall on Mary and Tom, as well as their family as they were the only ones left in that area.

During my recovery, I was sent to a rehabilitation home near our mobile home in North Port. Gene remained in our mobile home overnight, as a base of operations, but visited me usually at breakfast and stayed until dinner time. He brought his lunch for noon and ate at a table with me and two other very nice full-time residents. Our son-in-law, George, prepared dinner for Gene and brought it up in trips from Fort Myers. All Gene had to do was warm it up. The facility staff people were very helpful. The meals, while not gourmet, were very good, and they provided ice cream at the meals. The ice cream always made my day. I had physical and occupational therapy while I was there which helped with my stability. I also had breathing exercises, along with the other therapy, which I did not enjoy, but the aide who really liked me was good at encouraging me, in a diplomatic, but forceful way. She always called me Miss Mary, as did most of the other aides. She did that more often because I needed a lot of encouragement to complete the breathing exercise. I still had some of my senses, so I did not follow up her encouragement with a lot of anger. She was lucky.

George and Kathy, in the meantime, were on the hunt for a house for us to buy in the right price range near them. They found one they liked and had Gene take some time one day to travel with them to view it. The real estate dealer took George and Gene to a few houses before that for comparison purposes. When Gene saw the house that George and Kathy liked he fell in love with it. It was a two-bedroom with an office that could be used as a third bedroom if necessary and had large white tile floors in an open setting with lots of natural light. It also had all relatively new appliances and a large lanai overlooking a man-made lake, with a view of a fountain that lit up at night. Most of the furniture was also included in the price, which was part of the negotiation. The lanai was what really sold Gene on the house. He thought I would really enjoy sitting out there with a serene view of the lake and the water fountain that lit up at night. Unfortunately, by the time we got there, my Alzheimer's had progressed to the point that I had little incentive to do that, and Gene's dream did not meet reality.

We were not able to move into the house right away because the owners could not take occupancy in their new house in Naples, where the wife worked, for a few weeks. Since we had the mobile home to stay in, we agreed to have them stay in what was now our house, for a low rental price.

Before we left the mobile home, we were invited to a Canadian friend's home. They were very nice people who were renting the double-wide mobile home which Tom and Mary had bought and had refurbished. When we arrived there, I panicked at the three steps leading into the house, even though, I had been able to handle them on a prior visit. They saw a different side of me as Alzheimer's had taken over my mind. It had progressed significantly, in a short time. It was an embarrassing moment or two, but with the host's help, I was able to negotiate the climb.

In the meanwhile, George, who has a flair for good taste, had us buy two electric recliner chairs for the new house and he picked out pictures to go with the motif of the new house along with other items we might need, such as dishes, etc.

Back in Poughkeepsie, New York, our house remained vacant while Mary and Tom dealt with their work obligations. For our daughter Mary, it was getting ready for audits which included late nights working at home for her job as chief financial officer for the County Water and Waste Water Authority. For Tom, his job at IBM required late-night calls overseas, a few days a week, and his time chairing the Planning Board for the Village of Wappingers Falls. When the time became available, they went to the house and repaired things that mattered as well as organized the furniture to better stage the house for sales appeal. It was a lot of work, but they did a great job. The house was then put on the market with a real estate agent who did a fantastic job. The house was sold relatively fast, although we did drop the selling price during the negotiation to cover a new roof and a few other assorted things. We were pleased with the sale and the buyers were pleased with the house, even after they moved in.

Our car in Poughkeepsie also needed to be sold. Tom and Mary sold it back to the Honda dealer we had bought it from for us. In the meantime, we sold the mobile home in North Port at a lower price than the remodeling called for. Both houses were sold for less than we had hoped for, but we were rid of the taxes, etc. We had gained more than enough money to cover the cost of our new house in Fort Meyers.

Then came the problem. Since our new house came with most of the furniture, another job for Mary and Tom was to get rid of all the Poughkeepsie furniture. Most of it was sold at a low price, except a relatively expensive dining room set which was given to Habitat For Humanity. We had rebuilt the first floor to include a space for a washer-dryer combination so that it eliminated the need to go to the basement to wash clothes. Even though it was newer than the one in the basement, the buyers decided that they did not want to use them, so that had to be disposed of also. It was another hard job to clear the place in time for the new owners to move in, but Tom and Mary made it happen.

We finally got settled in our new Florida house in a community called Silverlakes. We were met by the community's official greeter, Shirley, who was originally from Missouri. She was very pleasant and knew that I had Alzheimer's. Shirley made a point of complimenting me on my outfits when she saw me at the community dinners. I guess Gene got something right in picking out colors that complement each other since this was not his specialty, to say the least. There I go again, belittling the poor guy, but as you know from my prior comments, I am brutally honest, and Alzheimer's did not help.

It was soon St. Patrick's day, and the corned beef was delicious at our first community dinner. With my Irish heritage, it was one of my favorite meals. Irish coffee was provided with the meal, and I naturally had Gene get a cup for me, even though in my later life, I was not a big alcohol drinker, except for a glass of Port wine. That was my father's favorite and I was accustomed to it. At the dinner, Shirley gave us take-home meals as well. Wow! What a bargain. This was repeated at the next dinner, by another person. Shirley probably suggested that. I guess that she felt sorry for Gene, or suspected his cooking may not have been gourmet. Gene was still learning how to cook, so I will let the answer to that be in the mind of the reader. That same neighbor still texts Gene to see how he is doing.

Gene always struggled to get the Rollator walker up the ramp to the clubhouse when I could not walk by myself. The walker, which is difficult enough to push on a level surface, was not designed to be pushed while someone sat on the seat, and was not recommended to be used that way. It was very difficult to push up an incline or over a ridge in the doorway with me in it. Our legs could clash at times so we had to be careful. As they saw us struggling, there was always a neighbor to help.

The Silverlakes community also has a free ice cream social for all ages. One year when they had money left over from the community breakfasts and dinners, they treated the community to a free Chinese dinner which one signed up for. The clubhouse was full.

When Gene got home from a couple of hospital visits after I passed away, one neighbor, originally from Rhode Island, brought over special soups. He still does. Other neighbors brought over desserts. Our friendly neighbor that had greeted us still makes sure that he gets desserts whenever she bakes them. Her husband drops them over at our house and Gene has become friendly with both of them. He also meets a friend when he walks in the morning and their chats make the walk seem shorter for both of them. What a great community! We are so fortunate to have spent some time there.

It may surprise the reader that it is not a senior community. It is so nice to see the children around the area and have such nice neighbors, regardless of age.

One of the things you learn in Florida is that you cannot tell if an out of the area call is a nuisance call, a neighbor, or even a doctor's office. We received calls or texts from locals with area codes of Hawaii, Missouri, and New York from home health aides, as well as neighbors, etc. We even got a call from a doctor's office labeled from Russia.

Gene's role in Florida was increased to not only cook and maid work, but he also was a full-time valet and caregiver. In the beginning, I was still able to walk with the use of my walker in the house, and a four-wheel Rollator walker with a seat built in, when we were going to a store or the doctor's office. My ability to walk any distance eventually diminished and Gene had to push me full time when we went anywhere using the Rollator walker. He pushed me out to the stores, doctor's visits, and church.

Since I could not stay home alone, Gene would position me just inside the entrance of the Publix grocery store near our new home while he shopped. I must have attracted the attention of the manager, or one of the employees, because a cart for handicapped adults who could not drive an electric cart, appeared on the scene. It was similar to a child seat cart and I sat facing Gene. It was great since I had company and Gene could ask me if I wanted certain items. One of the cashiers commented on how great an idea it was. Kudos to whoever brought it to the attention of the Publix grocery store manager.

At this stage, I was now in what Gene called pull-ups, but often I would soak through them, and Depends were added. Later, when hospice took over, I graduated to adult diapers. They were much more efficient. Much of the problem was that I waited too long to use the bathroom. I was always content to stay still. Content is another one of those diplomatic words.

Initially, we attended a large Catholic Church near us and I could sit in my walker at the rear of the Church during Mass. They had a beautiful choir, and since I had sung in a public choir in New Bedford, I thought I would join. The choir sat on the altar in plush seats facing the attendees. The first rehearsal seemed to go well and I was pleased. However, I had to have help going up the small number of steps to the choir seating area. Gene was worried that since I had a tendency to wet myself that I may have stained the plush seat covers. That was not the case. Gene noticed that at times I had my eyes closed and my mouth open when the rest of the choir was singing. Having my mouth open was getting more characteristic as my Alzheimer's progressed. When my mouth was open, it was a strange slanted shape, as if I had a recent stroke. But it was the way I usually looked with the disease when I slept or was in my quiet mode.

Easter Sunday was on the horizon with a big performance for the choir. The choir director called the house and talked to Gene. He had noticed my behavior and felt that it would be best for me to sit out the Easter Mass. Gene agreed and suggested that it might be best for me to sit in one of the pews even during rehearsals so that I could practice with the choir without disturbing anyone. I literally blew my stack when he told me. Even though Gene told me that it was his idea and not the director's. I refused to accept that. I still blamed the choir director, saying that he was discriminating against an Alzheimer's patient. I remained adamant about talking to the pastor about this, but Gene decided that we would start attending a Catholic Church further away from our house instead. He felt that it was the best solution to avoid an embarrassing situation.

The new Church was smaller but very nice. The entrance to the Church was sloped up and Gene had to push the walker up while entering and keep it from rolling too fast going down. It was also difficult for Gene to hear since we sat on a bench at the rear of the Church. I had to be helped onto and off the bench since my stability was worsening. The situation became much better when we purchased a transport chair. Gene had not purchased one earlier because someone told him they were unstable, but he finally had to resort to one. Gene had always been reluctant to get a full wheelchair. They were difficult to maneuver in our house and he had heard of an Alzheimer's patient losing use of his legs, probably from not using them. He did not want that to happen to me. I could not have wheeled myself for any distance at that point anyway. For the brief time we had to use the transport chair, we both enjoyed it better than the walker. It was a lifesaver in many ways. I could stay sitting in it during Mass and Gene did not have to work as hard to push it, or get tangled in my legs. It was also easier to put the transport chair in the car trunk since it easily could be folded into a smaller profile. We had bought a new car for the safety features, but we also needed space in the trunk for the walker, so we bought a full-sized car. We could have easily bought a smaller car if we had a transport chair from the start. Timing is everything.

Gene Damm

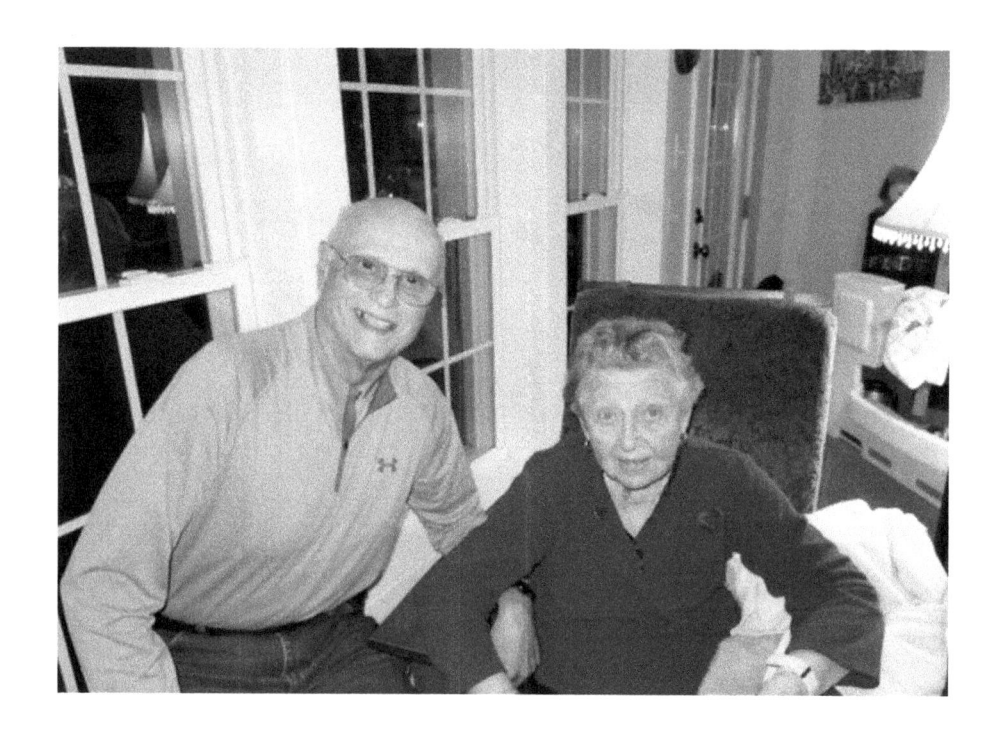

In The Eyes of an Alzheimer's Patient

The Beginning of the End

As the Alzheimer's progressed, the choir issue was forgotten, and we moved back to the Church nearer to home. But then COVID-19 hit, and we reverted to watching mass on television. I say we, even though Gene was never sure, with my closed eyes, how much I was absorbing. When the pandemic was in full swing, and we were isolated except for doctor's appointments, Gene would call people and have me talk to them. That was enjoyable, but eventually, I, who was usually very talkative with friends, stopped talking, and Gene had to take over the conversation.

I was increasingly losing my ability to control my legs to walk, but Gene still felt he could take care of me by himself. This is a mistake that many caregivers make, which too often leads to their demise, prior to the patient's demise. I had fallen in the house a few times as my balance and strength were giving out. One time George had to come over and help me off the floor. The other was a more serious fall coming out of the shower, and the EMTs had to come to help me up. Gene was unable to pick me up and called 911. It was an embarrassing situation as I was unclothed. Fortunately, my mind was not working properly, and I did not notice.

I was slipping faster than Gene thought would happen, and the change in me was becoming more apparent. Even when I was able to use the walker in the house, I insisted that Gene follow behind me day and night as I walked to the bathroom. If I felt that he wasn't as close as I wanted him to be, I panicked.

At one point, the family council decided that Gene needed a house cleaner to assist with the basic home cleaning. Gene compromised on it being every other week. In the meantime, Gene was concentrating on helping me shower and getting me dressed. I was becoming more disabled as time went on. Gene's bleeding ulcer acted up, and he needed to be hospitalized. To help with my needs, the family council convinced Gene to bring in a 24/7 caregiver while he was away. The cost was almost $4,000 for the few days, but it had to be done. Gene was back in the hospital again shortly after that, and the process repeated itself.

Most of the aides were very good and took good care of me. The only exception was one aide who appeared not to be familiar with assisting an Alzheimer's patient or what her responsibilities as a full-time aide were. Kathy noticed this and called the office to request that she not come back. Unfortunately, they had to keep her on the next day. When Gene returned from the hospital, he saw the picture that was presenting itself. He had to call her in from the lanai to assist me. When I did not want to take a shower, she yelled at me and finally resorted to a sponge bath. When she left, Gene called the office himself and reiterated that we did not want her to come again. The issue was closed with no question of her coming again despite their staffing problems.

I always wanted to delay or not shower for other aides because of this bad experience. Thankfully, I never got yelled at again. Not even when my nighttime incontinence required an early morning cleansing. Most of the aides were able to convince me or tell me to take a shower, without getting into a fight about it. However, it did take a while to get to that point and there was a time when one aide left at the end of her shift without showering me, rather than fighting with me. That made it more difficult for Gene.

In The Eyes of an Alzheimer's Patient

Gene was beginning to get quite tired, and I started to need even more assistance. The decision was made by the family council that I should continue to have additional help with showering and dressing to take more of the burden off Gene. I keep using the term family council to try to be diplomatic, rather than using Gene's words that, with three daughters, he had three other bosses. When I was alive, he said that he had four. He always said that the girls took care of their father. His life was saved several times by their insistence that he be taken to the hospital. I might add that they also did the same for me. Little did Gene know that I would remain the fourth "boss" from his love for me.

When the aides came in the morning, Gene had laid the clothes out for me to wear, including the special briefs and Depends. He also instructed the aides about my breakfast and he laid out the food to give me. Since their minimum time was four hours, Gene, who still thought that he could take care of me himself, was upset that some of the aides would just sit for the rest of their allotted time. Gene had always said that the housework was of less concern than working with my mind to keep it active. Gene was not happy that some of the aides did not do that. Some of them would do light housework and talk to me. Those were the good ones. One even tried to play games with me. I played for a little while, but I did not like games, and my eyesight was failing me, even with the large piece Alzheimer's puzzle that Gene had bought for me. I finally got them to stop with the games and puzzles. It was very frustrating to pay for four hours of work where most of the time, a number of them were sitting down while I was in my silent mode. That was all right for 24/7 care, but with Gene home, it was unacceptable to him. Since he preferred to feed me my breakfast and lunch, they did not have an awful lot of physical work to do, except bathe me.

He shifted the aides from five days a week to three days a week, which was a compromise with the family council. He had already been taking full care of me on the weekends, so he figured a break every other day during the week was good enough to reduce his burden. That may have been a mistake. Gene still handled the household chores. The man who had everything done for him, by me and his secretaries, often bemoaned the fact that when they invented fitted sheets, they should have required that they be marked to show which was the top and which was the bottom. In his early attempts to make the bed, it was like circling the wagon train as he twisted and turned it to find the right fit.

Gene eventually found a more acceptable agency with nurse's aides better matched for my needs. The COVID-19 pandemic impacted the aide's ability to come to the house, and Gene's workload increased again. Unfortunately, I was now becoming more challenging to handle.

Gene had volunteered to do swim stroke coaching for a half-hour, one day a week, for the Swim Florida swim team. I had encouraged him to do that and more despite my illness. He would take me to the pool and meets, in my walker, and I would sit there waiting for him to finish. The head coach was not only a great coach but was also a great person in that he cared for his swimmers. He would also take time to come over and talk with me. For the half-hour, he decided what stroke he wanted Gene to work on with the best swimmers in that stroke. Coach Mac and Gene got along fabulously, and he always showed appreciation for Gene's effort. Unfortunately, COVID-19 put an end to that.

In The Eyes of an Alzheimer's Patient

The Further Crumbling

I was beginning to experience what is called, "Sundown Syndrome." Although it usually occurs at night or late afternoon, I slept so much that I experienced it in the daytime as well. Sundown Syndrome affected me through hallucinations and disorientation. Nighttime was the most traumatic for me and for Gene. I began having hallucinations of people being in the lanai that caused me to get his attention. Some of the symptoms, of Alzheimer's, in addition to hallucinations, are sudden mood swings, screaming, more confusion than normal, even anger and aggression, among others. If the patient can walk, they might pace. It pays to keep doors securely locked at night, and not just to keep people out. You do not want the patient to be roaming the streets alone. They might also try to drive a car to somewhere they knew, for no known reason. I was not a walker, so that was one thing that Gene did not have to worry about. He did guard our car keys as a precaution. Sleep was still at a premium at night, and when I got his attention to come talk to the guests I believed were there, or he heard me talking about them, his sleep would be interrupted. He usually has trouble staying asleep anyway, and this added to his difficulties.

In the daytime, I would also talk to people who were not there, and Gene would just agree with me or say something innocuous to keep me comfortable and not get upset. Several times, I reverted to telling Gene that we needed to work on relays for the college meets. He would just agree with me. One time I even recognized that I was really talking to a fictitious person. That bit of sanity was a surprise. He had a little help in taking care of me at night when my daughter from Oregon was there, but even then, Gene took his turn. In his mid-80s, this did not bode well for his health. It was not good for my daughter, either who had to be well-rested to work remotely during the day. My hallucinations were not just of other people. I envisioned that I had made dresses for all my great-granddaughters, and told that to everyone I talked to. One of our grandchildren even believed I might have made them until their mother said it was not real.

I had a fear of tight clothes, so Gene had the job of making sure that the things I wore were loose. Some Alzheimer's patients feel the need to shed their clothes. I sometimes did as well. Gene would find me in the chair, with my blouse off, and nothing underneath it, or over me. He was terrified that someone might come and see me from our lanai. Gene would quickly help me get dressed again.

I was reaching the stage where I was getting incontinent with both urination and bowel movements. Cleanup of both me and the house was challenging for Gene. Fortunately, we had tile floors throughout the house. As much as it was a challenge to clean up tile floors, it would have been impossible with rugs. A number of times, he had to clean me, the bathroom, as well as the floors. Gene got upset at me a couple of times, but realizing that I could not help myself and that it was wrong to get angry, he started to react in a more calming way. My yelling did not help either one of us, especially Gene. Holding back on getting upset and not retaliating to any anger issues also did not help his ulcer. While Gene did the laundry, I would fold the clothes as he knew I liked to do. I had even mentioned that to him, as a way of helping. In between washings, he would take clothes from the bedroom for me to fold. He knew that they would be moved from one pile to the other without being folded, but it kept me busy. He wouldn't have folded them anyway. He was definitely not the neatest person with respect to clothes. Excuse me, Gene, for pointing that out, but you know I like to speak the truth. Gene needed to get additional help but did not want people sitting in our house overnight, waiting for an event to happen. He felt the daytime support, which he renewed with another agency, was sporadic at best in keeping me occupied. Extension of the daytime support of this type was not a good option in his mind, but it was our only option.

Gene Damm

And Then Came Martha

In a previous conversation, when Gene was looking for a senior gathering, they mentioned that we might be eligible for respite care provided by the state of Florida. Since they did not have anyone available at the time, Gene thought that it was long forgotten. About the time that I was getting worse and having trouble staying awake during the day, the center called and said that an aide named Martha was available. She was the best thing that happened to both of us during my disease. Martha was a former nurse with the patience of a Saint. She came to sit with me from 2-6 PM Monday through Friday.

Gene knew that I did not like games, but I used to like crossword puzzles. Martha would sit, with a calming voice, and patiently ask me what a clue or word meant and to the surprise of both Gene and Martha, I would usually very quickly come up with the word. They had found a key to an undestroyed part of my brain. In came the crossword puzzles from the Internet and Dollar Tree. They were just right for me. Martha also played a music channel on the television since music is often a key to the brain of an Alzheimer's patient while we were working the puzzles. She also got me to talk about my past life and got me to ask about her life. I really enjoyed our time together. She was a friend, as well as a companion. When Gene would be away at an appointment, I sometimes had a bowel movement and had to be cleaned and changed. She was very calm about it. If Gene was taking me somewhere, she made sure that she changed my clothes to something that looked presentable. When I was able to get to the table for dinner, as part of my exercise, she would get me there before she left. She even brought me some sippy cups she found in the children's area of the local grocery store because she thought they might be better, and they were. They were almost impossible to spill, as opposed to the ones that we had bought prior to that. She accomplished what the other aides had not, and found a path to working with my brain. This was a relief to Gene. Many times he had asked the prior aides to assist me in this manner, but they never did. Martha worked with the part of my brain that would work, and pulled it into the present, despite other parts being destroyed in processing information correctly.

If I wanted to rest for a while, she kept busy doing things around the house. She even arranged the clothes in Gene's bureau. Gene remarked that it was so neat that even his Tee shirts looked like they were ironed. This was quite a change from Gene just tossing them in the drawer. One day, she decided that my side of the closet was too cluttered, and she packed away all the off-season clothes for storage. A few days later, Gene noticed that the clothes she had taken down were in plastic bins. He had not remembered that number of bins left over from the shipment from our New York home. Gene then asked her where she got them. The answer was "Lowes." Gene responded, drawing out her name, "Maaaarthaaaaa, how much did you pay for them?" Her reply was five dollars for each. Gene immediately paid her for them.

At Christmas time, we sent her a gift basket from Costco for all the work she had done with me. She was very thankful, and even though we did not want a return gift, the next time she came, she brought a beautiful poinsettia plant for us. After I passed away, Gene wanted to keep the custom up of remembering her. He had a talk with her, stating that he was not going to do it if she returned with a gift for him. Fortunately, it worked out. This was Gene's way of thanking her for all the comfort she willingly gave me. I do not know how many "Marthas" there are in this world, who have both compassion and work ethic, but we were blessed by having one. Mother Teresa would have been well pleased with her. Martha will always live in our family's memories. We can only hope that there are more "Marthas" in this world to bring back more life to the brain of other Alzheimer's patients and provide needed relief to the patient's primary caregiver.

In The Eyes of an Alzheimer's Patient

Gene Damm

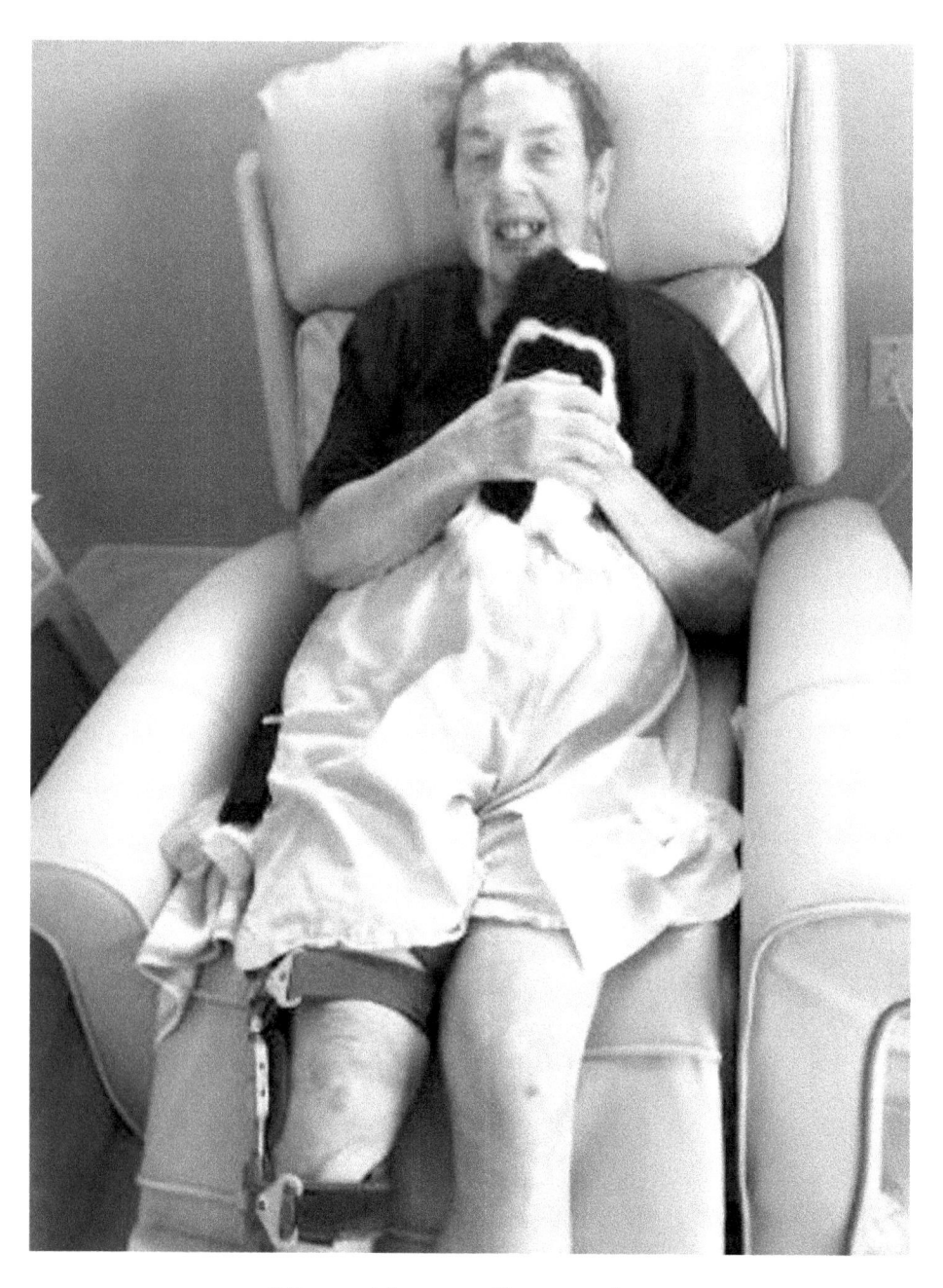

Mary with one of her toy dogs

In The Eyes of an Alzheimer's Patient

The Beginning of the Final Stages

I was starting to lose my appetite at the table and even in my recliner chair, which eventually had become my eating area as well as my bed since my legs constantly gave out on me. When I decided that I did not want to eat, George would bring over dishes that I usually liked, and I would eat again for a while. He even brought over Portuguese Kale Soup, which my father used to make. I loved it and used to make it for our family. However, that did not last long as my appetite failed. Gene even tried to feed me by hand, so I would at least have something nourishing. My eyesight was fading as the Alzheimer's increased, so I would often try to use my hands to pick up my food. A person looking in from the outside would think that I was eating like an animal.

Once, Kathy and George decided to bring Easter dinner, which we could eat together. For some reason crowds, even small ones, can affect an Alzheimer's actions. I decided not to eat. Eventually, I was 24 hours without food and little to drink. By night time, I was totally drenched and still refused to get up. Gene finally said that if I did not get up to at least change, he would have to call EMS to take me to the hospital. That convinced me to get up. When I got up, my clothes and the protective pad on the chair, were like wet rags. Once I was changed into dry clothes and the pad replaced, I did eat a little something. I used to like to snack on grapes and pretzels, so that was the natural thing to offer me before I went back to sleep. It had been a tough day for everybody, especially for Gene.

At another time, Mary and Tom thought that it would be a good idea to have their children, grandchildren, and Tom's mother come to see me in Florida before I got much worse. Kathy and George and their family joined the group at our place for dinner which George had prepared and brought over. The hope was that my grandchildren and great-grandchildren might see me once more, before my situation got much worse. Unfortunately, that kind thought was dashed. I was past that point. Alzheimer's did not want me to enjoy myself and I sat in my chair not eating at the table and being unsociable. It was another case of Alzheimer's affecting one's mind with crowds, even with those I loved dearly.

I also had trouble remembering names and got aggravated when people asked me the question of who they were, to see if I recognized them. It was one of my temper issues which Alzheimer's can trigger. It assisted my somewhat already bipolar personality. Only now I did not change to a loving person again, who forgot the altercation. I just succumbed to the solitary confinement that is customary with Alzheimer's. There were times when the paid aides were present in the house that I would get furious at them, but when they were about to leave, I did not want them to go. One of them told Gene that I did not like her. He laughed and told her about the last time this had happened, and sure enough, the pattern repeated itself.

In The Eyes of an Alzheimer's Patient

Reality is Faced

As my doctor began to recognize that the disease was overtaking me, he suggested, at one of my visits, that Gene should consider hospice for me. This was the same doctor, who when I said that I liked his tie in my earlier stage, deliberately wore different ties for my visits until he said that he ran out of them. He was the doctor who laughed when he asked me if I sat in the recliner with my legs level with my heart, and I responded, "What do you want me to do stand on my head?" He used to laugh at my other remarks also during my visits. Each time I wisecracked, Gene was overjoyed because it was a sign that I was in a good mood, being my natural self, despite the Alzheimer's.

Gene turned hospice down at this point in time. He knew several times I had looked like I was soon to leave this earth, but I had recovered. He also felt that I did not meet the traditional six months guideline for eligibility. My doctor acquiesced and did not push the issue. He considered it Gene's decision but brought it up in a future visit when I had further deteriorated.

Gene asked him at that visit, in a discrete way, that he hoped that I would not understand, about the six months guideline. The doctor's answer was, "It is not out of the question." Gene interpreted that it meant that I would meet the guidelines, and this time agreed to follow the doctor's recommendation. Gene may never forget that moment, even though he was unsure of whether that was a good call. As it turned out, it was exactly the right time for that type of assistance. My doctor was right, as usual.

Hospice visited us and agreed that I did need help. They arranged for a nurse's aide to come in to bathe me seven days a week with a nurse coming in once a week to assess my medical needs. This by itself took some of the load off Gene. They managed the medicine that they were responsible for, and provided refills, and new medicines as needed.

The main nurse assigned to us was a woman named Valerie. She was extremely helpful and always ready to be on call. Gene was very impressed with how much empathy she had even being an outsider. She was also very professional in dealing with us. And I do mean us. She was concerned about Gene, as the caregiver, as well as me as the patient.

She checked on me and my medication needs during her weekly visits and answered calls when the family was wondering about several issues. The hospice nurse's aides were also nice and able to get me to bathe without the usual argument on my part, which was a tribute to the way they handled me. They really knew how to communicate with an Alzheimer's patient, although each in a slightly different way. I convinced them to brush my hair, which was not part of their job. Gene knew from watching prior, non-hospice aides, that brushing my hair could be used as a motivation to get me to do what they needed done. I always enjoyed my hair being brushed and used to ask my children, my grandchildren, and great-grandchildren to brush it for me.

Hospice even visited on weekends if my blood pressure was off, or if I had oxygen issues. The nurses always said that the family should not be afraid to call them if something was worrying them. During a visit, when my oxygen level was low, they decided that I needed an oxygen unit. They called it in, and shortly after that, an oxygen unit came to the house, at no cost to us. We were told by one of the nurses who examined me, that regardless of what the oxygen meter showed, I should get oxygen if my lips were turning blue. They were so good at coming out. Even when my blood pressure dropped and they knew it was probably not alarming, they came to make sure. Hospice even provided a volunteer aide a couple of times when Gene had a doctor's appointment.

One time, a weekend hospice nurse was evaluating me and asked who the president was, I said, "Harry Truman." She followed it with a question about what year it was and I said, "1957." Since it now was the year 2020, I had failed the test, but neither Gene nor the nurse commented on it. This was not new with me, but it was getting worse. I did seem to remember Gene, but not much else.

During one of Valerie's early visits, I was really in bad shape and it looked like, in hospice words, that I was transitioning. It was the kind way of saying that there was a possibility that I would pass away in the near future, and it might be good to have the family there. In the end, it turned out, as it did at later times, that I recovered, but the visits did allow the family to see me again. Fading so low and then recovering to a better level was one of the reasons that Gene felt that hospice would sooner or later remove my eligibility for their service. Fortunately, they did not. My doctor's timing was close to perfect.

Valerie was very comforting to me. She treated me as though I was her own mother. I cannot say enough good things about her as a nurse and a caregiver. In addition to the aides bribing me with brushing my hair, as I mentioned earlier, she also would brush my hair to comfort me. She told Gene that hospice provided an opportunity for me to be looked after for five days in one of their Hospice House facilities. It was a free service as a five-day respite for the caregiver, but Gene, at that point, did not want me to be away if it could be avoided. Here again, it turned out that Valerie was right in her assessment of the burden on Gene, and was telling him in so many words that it was advisable. This was not the first time he was wrong in assessing how much he could do, but at his age, and with his health issues, it was not smart. He was lucky that he avoided the fate of many a caregiver and was around to be with me when I passed. We also had a non-denominational spiritual leader from hospice come at times to talk and comfort me, never mentioning my near death. It was a nice touch for them to have a spiritual leader in their repertoire. They, of course, had to have consent from my family for him to visit. Gene readily agreed.

When Gene was in the hospital one time, and I was not doing well, the family council decided that going to the Hospice House might be good for me. It provided me with 24-hour medical assistance, and they were able to try to revive me. Strange how that worked, but it followed the pattern of looking like it was the end and then reviving. Their friendly way, and the companionship they provided, pulled me out of my slump. They fed me well, managed my medicines, and periodically came into the room to care for me. The volunteer aide that stayed with me to allow Gene to leave for his own medical appointments worked out of the same Hospice House where I was admitted. She also visited me there. Then she called Gene at the hospital to report to him on how I was doing. How is that for caring? She truly matched the title of caregiver.

I was still in the Hospice House when Gene got out of the hospital, and Mary brought him to see me. She also brought replenishing snacks for me. Gene was suitably impressed, but still not sure if we would need to use Hospice House again once he was home to take care of me. Wrong again.

During the pandemic, Martha was told that she should not continue the visits, but as conditions eased, she was thankfully able to come back. She continued to visit me up until the point that I went to the Hospice House for the last time. With both hospice home care and Martha, the strain on Gene became a lot less, though his fears for both of us increased. The chain of events had already started a strain on his health.

There were other issues for Gene shortly after I passed away. These included two angina attacks which the medical professionals could not control with blood thinners. These episodes resulted in him needing surgery to enlarge and replace an old, now 95% blocked stent. They reluctantly did not replace it after the first angina attack, because he was on blood thinners as a result of a blood clot they found during the first angina attack.

Gene had some bleeding issues on the blood thinners so they performed a colonoscopy and removed part of a polyp to do a biopsy. Although it came out negative, a clip that they had put in at the time to close the wound, fell out a week or so later. It had landed on an artery. This was not good when he was on two blood thinners as a result of his blood clots and heart issues. After extreme blood loss and an emergency nighttime operation, the gastroenterology doctor said that he had lost a bucket of blood.

I say the following for the benefit of all caregivers. With the strain it takes to provide ongoing care, even an unrelated health incident can all too often take an overworked caregiver out of this world before their loved one. That is not uncommon, which is why various groups have respite sessions for them. Those of you who may be experiencing a similar situation, please think seriously about this warning. Do not do what Gene did. He was lucky and survived because he always stayed in some modicum of shape. Even though I was gone for a short while before the angina attacks, it is another reminder that the life of an older caregiver has its own risks. Trying to do everything by themselves, without respite time, can be dangerous.

Gene Damm

My Final days

I was slipping fast into the stage of complete helplessness. I was not eating, I could not walk, and talking was challenging. Trying to assist me when I had difficulty standing up, or stopping myself from falling in the house was a challenge, to say the least. It was especially stressful for Gene after he had a pacemaker put in. He could not lift anything heavy with one arm. Trying to lift and steady me with one arm was both difficult and worrisome. At one point, he thought that I was falling when he went to get me out of the chair and would need to call George or 911 again for assistance. Fortunately, he was able to manage the event without hurting himself. One of the problems was that as the Alzheimer's progressed, instead of cooperating with the person lifting, I pushed down and resisted the help to lift me up because I feared that I might fall.

Cheryl was the nurse's aide on duty the day that Alzheimer's almost completely took over my system. There was no way I was getting up to shower. She then wanted to put me into the hospital bed, that hospice had provided, so she could sponge bathe me. I had always refused to go into that bed, but by this time my mind was so far gone that I offered no resistance. Cheryl then turned to Gene, whom she knew had the recent pacemaker installed, and said in no uncertain terms, "And you are not to try to get her up." It was very forceful, and my youngest daughter laughed at Cheryl. Cheryl knew how to handle both me and Gene. All my hospice aides were nice, but Cheryl had a commanding way about her. She was already well liked and this action further endeared her to the family council. It was then that everyone, including Gene, decided that I needed to go to Hospice House again. In Gene's mind this would help me recuperate to a more manageable state. It was a nice thought, but I was never to return to our house.

The Hospice House that I went to this time was in Fort Myers. It was relatively new and in a beautiful area with a man-made lake with several fountains, one of which was almost directly in back of an enclosed lanai attached to my room. I of course could not take advantage of the lanai, but it was a nice touch for patients who could. The room was large with the addition of a recliner chair and a built-in sofa arrangement, which could serve as a bed for family members. The sofa was not a comfortable bed, but it was a bed.

Erin, my nurse daughter from Oregon, came in to town and stayed overnight with Gene, one in the recliner chair and one on the sofa bed arrangement. I was not eating at the time, and eventually I was not able to take any liquids by myself. Liquids now had to be given to me via a syringe while massaging my jaw to help me to swallow. The spiritual leader for that Hospice House stopped by and he happened to be a deacon in a nearby Catholic Church. He administered the blessing of the sick to me, and Holy Communion to Gene and my son-in-law George, who were with me at the time. Prior to that, while I was at home, the pastor at our local church had given me a general absolution over the phone. I was at peace with the world, as I was almost ready to leave it.

When the five days of respite care was ending, Gene knew that it would still be necessary for me to stay there longer. He was concerned about the fees for this service and could not believe, after our prior experiences with other groups, how little they charged. It was a comfort to know that the beautiful room with its large lanai, the food service, and excellent nursing were not an issue. Gene was thankful for the wonderful nurses who were not only administering my medicine, but also changing my position in bed to provide comfort and prevent bed sores, even though they knew I was nearing the end.

Gene still hoped that I would last longer, but at the same time realized that I was no longer able to be taken care of at home. He made arrangements with the administrator to stay after my five days of respite care were over. I lasted only two days longer.

George joined Gene at my room during visiting hours before Erin arrived from Oregon. George and Erin tried their best to get responses from me, even if they were muted.

Gene had told Mary and Tom that they should wait to come until he was sure that my condition was critical and he would have a report in a day or two. He was not sure of what the outcome might be and did not want them coming again for a false alarm. This was his standard answer regardless of whether he or I was sick. This time his advice was fortunately ignored, since they were already packed and leaving. They did not tell Gene, giving him no choice. Kathy and George had indicated to the family that the end was closer than Gene wanted to believe. As in sports, that was a good call, since they otherwise may have missed my last hours. Mary and Tom drove from Wappingers Falls, New York, and joined George and Kathy staying overnight in one of the community rooms as things looked imminent. Erin and Gene were still staying in my room. The family was later told that staying overnight in the community room like this was not permitted and that they would need to come back during the daytime. They were also told that only two people at a time were permitted in the patient's room. The family knew about the two-person limitation, but wanted to be around if I passed during the night. They hoped that staying in the lounge might satisfy the two persons in the room rule, but accepted the management's ruling.

That part of the family, after hearing the rule, went to George and Kathy's house for a shower and to recuperate a little. There were no signs of a worsening of my condition. Erin and Gene remained as the two allowed people in the room. I looked asleep as usual. Then about noon, the nurse came in and told Gene that my skin was becoming mottled, which was a sign that my passing was near. Gene asked for a rough time estimate of our remaining time, and was told that it was anticipated within the next 72 hours.

Erin had stepped out to get some sandwiches at the little deli down the corridor, and Gene informed her what he was told when she arrived back at the room. They then stepped out to the lanai to eat. It was easier to talk and make calls there so as not to disturb me. Gene then called the rest of family to inform them of this latest information.

Erin had finished her sandwich first and went back in to see me. She did not see me breathing and immediately informed the nurse's station outside my room. The nurse came in, and confirmed Erin's observation. I had passed away. While the estimate the nurse had made earlier was the longest that I could last, no one expected it to be that soon. The family was informed that the limitation on visitors was now suspended and that the whole family could enter the room for as long as they needed to pay their last respects. It was July 27, 2020 at the age of 85, that I left this world.

A while before this last day, Gene was convinced by one of the family councils, to make funeral arrangements. Mary and George had talked to the funeral home earlier, and were key figures in ensuring that happened. They did a lot of checking on arrangements prior to discussing them with Gene, who pretty much was in denial and rejecting the possibility of my imminent death. Although he did see the sense in making arrangements for both of us. I had never wanted to discuss burial plots and what went with them. Based on prior talks, Gene knew better than to bring the subject up. It was similar to my earlier thinking that going to a doctor would mean that I had something seriously wrong. He, more than I, was resigned to our ultimate death, but preferred not to bring the subject up during my illness. Sane minds prevailed again, and he succumbed to our children's request to make the arrangements.

George and Gene had met with the funeral director to settle on the final procedures and cost, as well as the casket in which my remains would rest. Those arrangements had made it much easier for Gene when it actually happened. The Hope Hospice people took care of calling the funeral home for the family.

After my passing George, Tom, and Gene met with a funeral director to finalize arrangements, and pick out the stone for our grave. A beautiful blue stone with white lettering was selected and one of the funeral directors later said that it was the stone that he took people to see when they were trying to make final arrangements for their loved one. It was interesting to note that many longtime Floridians choose to have flat metal plaques as their grave markers. Gene did not know that at the time, but he would have chosen an upright stone anyway as I would have wanted a classic gravestone. The family council also decided that the statue I had of my favorite dog, a dachshund I named Rommel, should be buried with me. Rommel was a good dog, not afraid of man nor beast. He was good with the girls, although he was not one to play with them much. Our youngest daughter used to get on her knees and growl at him and he would growl back. But Rommel always made it known that he was definitely my and my elderly father's dog.

I must say that my funeral was a beautiful one. Both the church ceremony, and the burial were streamed live thanks to Tom, which allowed friends to view it. Only the immediate family were allowed into the church, and most of our friends were from out of town anyway, so the streaming was a great idea. Luckily our grandchildren from the west coast were able to attend. The priest performed a very nice homily and the flowers were beautiful. Some of our friends remotely cried at the ceremony which they also thought was beautiful. I really appreciate how strong our friendships were with our extended family.

The grave site was in a beautiful new area of the cemetery. It was a smaller area and had a beautiful dolphin fountain the family walked past on the way to the new home of my earthly body. The priest accompanied us to the site and said some kind words to the family members.

My grandson Chris, knowing I was about to pass away, had produced a special version of the hymn Amazing Grace that was played at the burial service. It brought tears to a lot of eyes, including viewers of the streaming, as they heard the emotion in his voice. The song link is: https://soundcloud.com/user-50462743. He graciously provided a free link to this song.

Among the people who spoke was Gene, who was still weak on his feet from his illnesses, and was using a cane. His sons-in-laws stood at each side him, at his request, ready to support him in the event that he collapsed due his shattered state and the talk he was giving.

I really appreciated that our wonderful family shared the burden with Gene for all the arrangements, and of course for what they did for him, before, and after my passing. They cared for both of us. Kathy and George still have Gene over for dinner most nights, unless they all go out to dinner. There is rarely a schedule conflict that prevents this. Erin visits him as often as she can, and Mary and Tommy always help him, when they are in Florida. They even took him to Disney World for a few days after my granddaughter's wedding. It was a real treat for him to see his great grandchildren from the northeast who were there enjoying the rides. Of course, everyone looks after him by phone. Our daughter Mary's mother-in-law, and our granddaughter' s mother-in-law were especially good at praying for both of us in our illnesses, and now they pray for Gene, as do one of our dear friends. We had prayers said at both church and synagogue. How can you miss?

George had visited our family doctor after my funeral and mentioned to him that my funeral had taken place. The doctor said, "I wish I had known. I would have been there." How is that for a doctor who had only known us for a little over a year? I guess he liked my quips when I was alert enough to give them.

We had a good life and the team of Gene and Mary, or Mary and Gene as I wrote on our cards to friends, survives in spirit. As I now live in a new world, I want to say God bless to everyone and hope that this book will help inform the readers on the effects of Alzheimer's on the patient and their loved ones, especially their caregiver.

You may ask why a person with my intelligence, and social capabilities, did not do more with my life. Gene thinks that in today's world, I could easily have been a corporate executive, or a school principal, which would have recognized my intelligence. However, given the choice, I would not change a thing about Gene's and my life together. I chose the path I followed with him, and it was all about the team, not us as individuals. His success was my success. I certainly loved my family and our swimmers, as well as all the friends we made along the way. I lived 85 good years, and though some of them were tough, I would not change a thing.

Please read the letters that follow. They will be enlightening of both my life, and other patients and caregivers, as well as the impact on family members. The impact on the family of a caregiver, and patient are described better than I could do.

God bless you all, and I leave with my favorite quote.

"Love is stronger than death"

In The Eyes of an Alzheimer's Patient

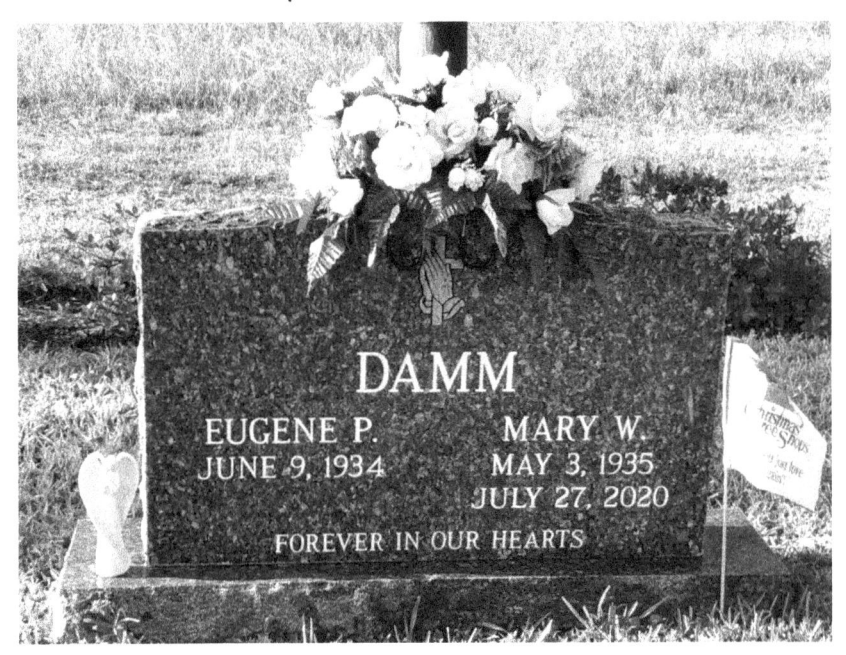

Mary's remembrance stone

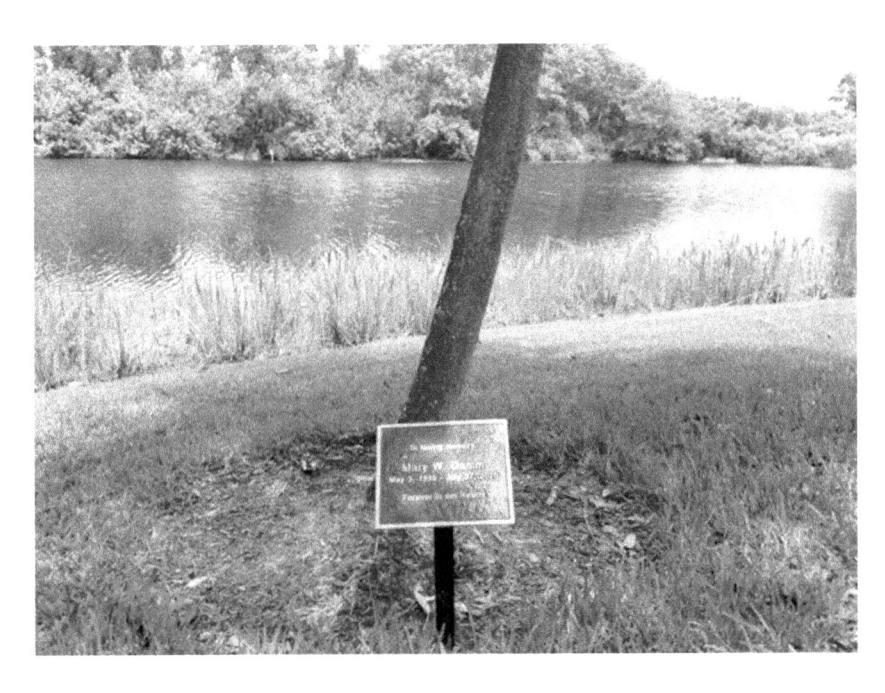

The Remembrance Plaque at Hospice House

Gene Damm
Family

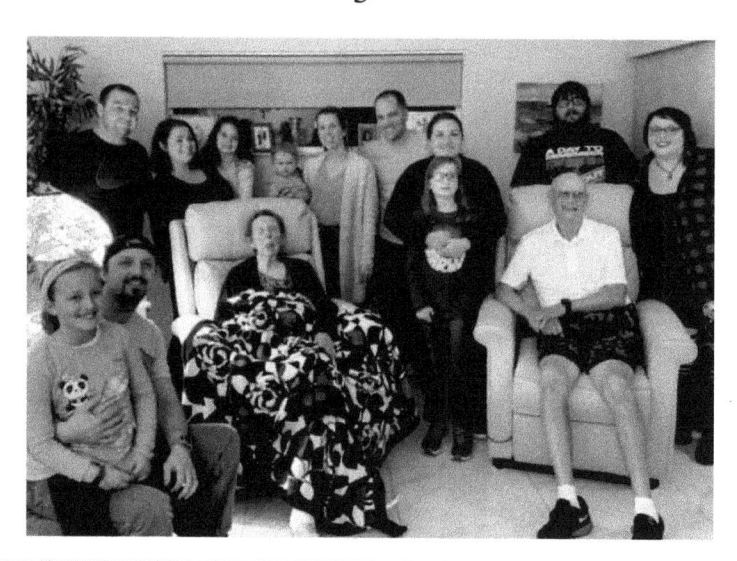

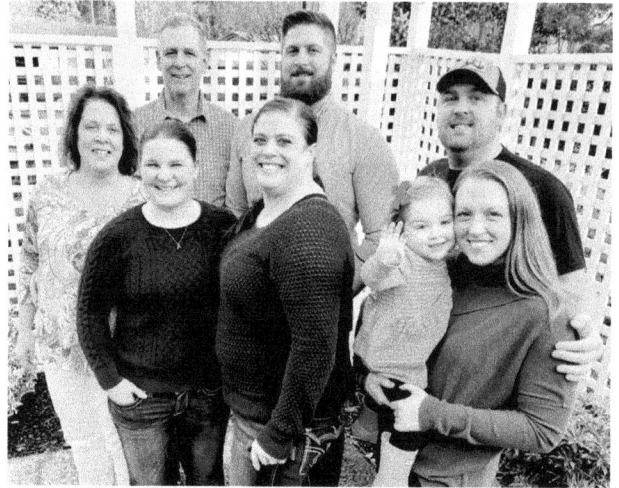

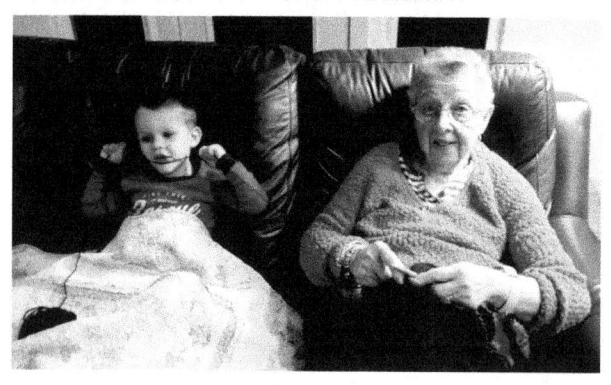

In The Eyes of an Alzheimer's Patient

The Plight of Others

Here are letters written by family members, friends, and caregivers describing their paths and struggles with either my Alzheimer's disease or their experiences with another loved one. I thank you for sharing your thoughts and all the love you have given me.

~~~~~~

A letter from our daughter, Mary Catherine

Probably one of the best words I could use to describe my mom's approach to life would be "engaged." She very rarely approached anything in half measures. She was involved in our activities as children and assisted and volunteered wherever needed. She followed her grandchildren's activities as well; and when great-grandchildren came along, she taught them little songs and read to them. She instilled in us an appreciation for our heritage. This involved not just our own personal background and of our ancestors that came to the United States through Ellis Island to build a better life for their family, but the whole concept of how lucky we were to be raised in this country, its history, and how important this was as part of our lives. Music appreciation was instilled in us frequently and to this day I can probably sing most Broadway show tunes from the 50s and 60s and many a patriotic song. Although graduating with honors from New Bedford High School, mom's family was not in a strong enough financial position to send her to college, and instead, she went to work to help support her family. She never gave up on her desire to pursue higher education and completed her Bachelor's Degree at the age of 57, majoring in English.

All these things and many others were a major force in her life and we found it hard to understand in the beginning why she was losing interest and not being as involved as she had been. She had overcome a lot of adversity in her earlier years in order to forge her achievements, supporting her parents as an only child and living with multiple phobias. She complained of being tired and just wanted to be "left alone." The family joke was that shopping was her sport and her hobby and that if we wanted her to keep close and follow us through Disney World, we could just use a shopping bag from one of her favorite stores as a flag on a pole in order to keep her focused on what direction we were taking. When her interest in shopping and her care in her appearance and hygiene began to decline, we knew there was a problem.

My grandmother (mom's mom) was diagnosed with Dementia back in the 1970s. It was very frustrating to my mom that my grandmother could just sit in a chair all day long, with no interest in conversation, people, food, etc. Although it was a different diagnosis and there are various stages of Alzheimer's, the result of withdrawing from the world around them was similar. And remembering how much it upset my mom to watch that, I often wondered how upset she would have been if she could see 20 years into her future. If possible, I think it would have been even more devastating to her than it was to her family to see this vibrant, embrace life with gusto personality, leave themselves behind to become part of a world that they struggle to break out of daily and their family and friends have a hard time breaking in.

~~~~~~

A letter from
Our daughter, Erin

I remember my mom in so many positive ways. She is remembered as mom, grandma, great-grandma, swim coach, mentor, and many more great things. She raised me to be respectful, kind, honest, strong, and independent. I spent quality time with her as often as I could, especially after we moved away for employment in the early 1990s.

It was very hard being away, especially after I started noticing changes, however so slight in her physical and mental status. She was reluctant to go to the doctors, as one of her several fears was a fear of doctors. In addition, she was of an age that feared the doctors would put her in a "home," if she was diagnosed with Alzheimer's. Thus, she hid her condition well, in the earlier onset of the disease, and on her good days, I even questioned the diagnosis of Alzheimer's myself.

Mom also had conditions that had similar symptoms to Alzheimer's, like decreased energy and loss of appetite. She had heart failure, diabetes, was blind in one eye, and could not see well out of her other eye. She had a stroke at one time, without an obvious permanent decrease in her mental/physical condition. Her gradual decline in energy and physical capabilities could have been a combination of her heart, kidney failure, increasing blindness, and/or Alzheimer's. Even her providers felt her heart failure, vision issues ,and/or her medications, including Digoxin toxicity, contributed to her mental and physical status changes.

Thus, it took an intervention by the doctors in Oregon, to get mom to move forward and see the provider that diagnosed her with Alzheimer's. They started with an occupational therapist evaluation and because of the results, asked her to follow up with a neurologist. We were finally getting some answers!

We took mom to the neurologist in Florida, who referred her for a neuropsychiatric evaluation, which occurred in January 2018. We explained to the neuropsychiatric provider that mom was forgetting to pay bills, not taking her medications correctly, calling my dog, by her deceased dog's name, not dressing as nice as she had in the past, and asking questions over and over again. She also withdrew from her favorite activities, like shopping. This evaluation was the turning point, for mom and dad. Having the Alzheimer's diagnosis and knowing mom was declining more and more helped my parents make some important decisions.

Dad had to take over the bills and we all had to learn not to get upset with mom. She could not help her behaviors. Her needs became more and more exhausting. She had to have her clothes picked out for her and needed assistance with her activities of daily living. Dad also had to cook all the meals, do the wash, and clean the house.

Alzheimer's escalated her fears and impacted her physical abilities and her ability to enjoy life, which caused her to be more and more homebound. Dad could no longer leave her alone.

I am grateful I had the opportunity to be with mom in the end. I spent 6-8 weeks caring for her and two of my biggest pleasures were listening to her answer crossword puzzle questions over and over again and taking her for a drive, to have ice cream. When I left after the first five weeks, she and I talked about me coming back to help care for her. That made my day!

Until she was nearing death, she knew my name. She clearly had Alzheimer's, but her heart gave out in the end. I fed her the last bites she ate, including her favorite chocolate ice cream a couple days before she passed. I spent the last two nights by her side. Mom is always in my heart.

~~~~~~

A letter from our daughter, Kathleen

Throughout my childhood, my parents always provided me with support. Mom took us where we needed to go and dad worked at his job and then coached us in swimming. They taught us to treat people with respect and to work hard in whatever we did. Mom was the caretaker during this time. When we all got married, they helped in whatever way they could, especially with our children. My kids would visit during the summer. Kasey during a college break went to Florida to visit and they took her to a Red Sox spring training game.

Gene Damm

As I remember, mom started to go downhill during the time Hanna, our youngest, was in college. Hanna would visit them often since she was close by. She would take my mom shopping and my dad would say don't lose her. Of course, I remember the day she did in the store and was calling us and my dad. She finally found her. Mom had just wanted to go to a different department.

We moved to Florida and only saw my parents when they were down for the winter. Then one year it became obvious she had Alzheimer's after being tested and the decision was made for them to stay in Florida. We found a house for them about 3 miles from ours. We would visit and bring food to them. That is when the tables turned and my dad became the caretaker.

He was getting rundown, made himself sick, and at that time help was brought in. Mom could remember a lot from her earlier years and especially getting ready for swim meets.

She loved George's cooking and would eat what he made even if she would say she didn't like it. She always remembered who George was.

She always wanted the best for her children, grandchildren, and great-grandchildren. The memories we all have are different and when together it is great to remember. She was happy to see Hanna was engaged. There was a time she said she made green dresses for us to wear, this was her in her mind. She never did.

On July 17, 2020, Hanna's birthday, she and I went there to visit. Mom said it was her own birthday and she was happy. That day she went to Hope Hospice. The nurse told my dad it was the best for both of them since he was not his best either. We went and saw her as much as we could. One day George called my sisters and told them to come down. With COVID it was difficult for all of us. We all were there to be able to say goodbye. It was the hardest for all of us to do. Alzheimer's is a disease that is not only tough for the patients but takes a toll on the caretaker and family.

We will never forget the memories we have of mom and what she gave us growing up and our children during their time with her.

~~~~~~

A letter from our oldest Granddaughter, Kimberly Lopez, with a Note from Her Daughter

When I think of grandma, there are so many memories. From lessons learned, to just "people watching" on a bench.

If you knew grandma, she loved to shop! She taught me how to have "an eye for a deal" and never have too much. I still can remember going shopping with her. Once she found a store she loved, that was the store you always went to. The two that stick out in my head are Kohl's and of course, the Christmas Tree Shop.

School was very important to Grandma. Report cards were reviewed every time and if you did well, you received a five-dollar bill out of Grandpa's wallet as soon as Grandma told him to give us money, haha! Reading was never my favorite thing to do, but Grandma always stressed the importance of it. I soon learned to love reading when Grandma bought me *Little Women* and from there wanted to read more.

Gene Damm

Grandma always told me to dress nicely when going out, no dungarees. I remember how she would iron everything. I don't iron nearly as much as Grandma did, but I learned that your clothes should look presentable. She also always picked out Grandpa's clothes. I think "Best Outfit" has to go to his plaid pants. They are the most talked about pants around!

A memory that I still can hear her saying is the infamous "Don't tell your Grandfather" when she would secretly pass us money when we would get together. Abigail now says that line and laughs every time.

Grandma loved Massachusetts. That is where she grew up and always wanted to share the history and love she had for it with us. When we were growing up, we would go to "the cottage." It was always Chris's favorite place, not always mine, but looking back I have some amazing memories from there. From swinging in the hammock, bathing in the lake when we lost power, taking walks around the neighborhood, and hearing the neighbor's dog, Bear, bark, or the smell of burnt toast waking us up and letting us know Grandma was up and ready for the day.

When Grandma would come over, it was like playing twenty questions. She wanted to know everything that was going on, from what you were learning in school to what you and your friends were doing. She always had some words of wisdom to share when we were telling her what was going on.

Christmas was Grandma's favorite holiday. You knew it was Christmas Day when Grandpa would walk in with many garbage bags filled with wrapped presents. And the rule was that you had to open presents one person at a time so that she could see. Christmas and Easter also meant that you would need a new outfit. You would get "holiday clothes" money to get a new outfit for Easter and Christmas Day. I still make sure we have something new to wear on both Easter and Christmas.

Sitting with Grandma was always fun. Before her dementia, she would just sit and people watch. When she wanted to get your attention to point something out, she would grab or pinch your arm. It usually was not politically correct, but usually always funny. One of the best things about Grandma was that she had no filter. If she was thinking it, she said it.

We would always joke with Grandma asking her who her "Favorite" was. If you ask Alberto, "Albertoes" as Grandma would say, he is the "Favorite," but there was always a battle between most of the grandkids and now with some of her great-grandkids. Abigail has put her name in the running. The battle of the "Favorite" is still going on to this day, but I know who her favorite was.

~~~~~~

A Letter From our Grandson, Christopher Morris with notes from his Daughters

I have been very fortunate in life to be able to say that I was given the opportunity to grow up having my grandparents around to be involved in my development and shape the person that I have become today.

Some of my earliest and fondest memories of my grandmother all begin the same way "out at the cottage" in Freetown, Massachusetts. I remember spending as much time as I could including weeks in the summer, just me and my grandparents. In August of 1991, Hurricane Bob struck the area, I was 8. I remember being nervous at the time but my grandmother made every effort to keep my mind occupied and assure me that everything would be OK. At night, she would rub my back and sit with me until I fell asleep. I remember her telling me stories of growing up in that area and things she and her friends used to do. That is something I have come to appreciate more as I have gotten older. This was a view into the person my grandmother was before she was my grandmother, her excitement and enthusiasm to teach me all about New England and its history has certainly stuck with me into adulthood. This area will always be a place that I feel closer to my grandmother and a place that I now take my family to as well, including one of her favorite places, the Whaling Museum in New Bedford, Massachusetts.

As a teenager, I became more aware of my grandmother's quick wit and infamous no filter speech, especially when it came to topics she thought were extremely important, such as education. I was far from the best student and did not even complete college. She made sure to let me know how she felt about my life decisions and even though she knew I may not like what she had to say, she was not afraid to tell me anyway. Her openness to speak her mind about anything or to anyone is something that I truly miss about her. Even on vacations to Disney World, my grandmother would not go on any rides, she would sit on a bench and strike up a conversation with whoever she could. At the time, I never did understand how she could enjoy this, but she really did find joy in just watching the rest of us have a good time. This was one of her simple pleasures in life.

This is a trait I try to stay conscious of in my own life. As the years passed and teenage years became adulthood, my grandmother was always a constant in my life. It was also unfortunately at this point that I started noticing small instances of memory loss with my grandmother. It started will small things we would joke about such as buying two of the same item for someone or forgetting to remove a price tag from a gift. It was also around this time I took over their lawn care and I would continue to do so for the next 10 years. Over time, it became less about the lawn and more about the time spent with them. This provided a good excuse to see my grandparents on a regular basis during a period of my life when I was starting a family and a career. This also allowed me to see changes in cognitive behavior on a closer level and some weeks were certainly better than others. A once sharp as a tack personality was not as sharp and it was becoming ever more apparent and upsetting. What I now know as one of the last months before the unplanned and permanent move to Florida, my family and I lived with my grandparents. This is a time I will always remember and cherish. Not only did I get to share space with them for an extended period of time, but my wife Nicole and our girls Madeline and Penelopy did as well. Though my grandmother was showing further signs of digression she was still aware of who we all were. She especially remembered all of her great-grandchildren who affectionately know her as "Mousey" for the game she would play with them. Over the course of the next year, we would talk and video chat regularly, though this was far from the same, we were grateful to still play an active role in her life. Not being able to be present for her became ever more difficult for me as time went on and I could not be there for her in her time of need, to comfort her as she did for me all those years ago at the cottage.

~~~~~~

Gene Damm
A Few Words from three of our Great Granddaughters

Abigail Lopez, age 8

Mousey always called me seaweed. She would always play with me. She had great taste in purses. I took some to remember her. I love her and miss her.

Author's note: During July fourth, almost a year from my wife's death, Abigail said, "Mousey was probably up there roasting marshmallows."

~~~~~~

Penelopy Morris Age 9

I loved Mousey. I remember last year we went to visit her and we had fun seeing her. We also took a family picture. I also remember we lived with them briefly. And I remember some nights we went to Olive Garden because it was Mousey's favorite. I also loved her warm, loving, caring, gentle smile.

~~~~~~

Madeline Morris Age 11

I loved Mousey. Mousey was funny and she loved watching old movies. Every time we were over at their house we would play with chalk and she would sit in a chair and watch us. It was very fun living with them for the time we did. We used to see them every week because daddy cut their lawn and we'd sit on the driveway and play. Mousey gave the best hugs and I loved to see her smile.

Author's note: The girls still wear pins from Mousey's collection in memory of her.

~~~~~~

In The Eyes of an Alzheimer's Patient
An Essay by our Great Granddaughter, Madeline Morris

"Thump." My backpack hit the ground like an elephant stomping on the dry savanna dirt.

"Girls, can you come here, we need to talk," my dad exclaimed urgently.

"OK!" my sister and I replied as I walked in. My parents' faces turned blue, as blue as the sky on a stormy day.

"What's wrong?" I ask. As I did so, my palms started to get sweaty and clammy at the same time. I also felt queasy and sick to my stomach.

"Well, sweety," my mother exclaimed to my sister and me, but in the softest voice possible, kind of like a whisper but louder.

As I sat on the couch, I wished the couch would just swallow me up, but it was just very squishy and soft. My parents start talking. All that I can think about are the possibilities of what the conclusion of this conversation will be.

When I focus on my parents, I finally hear the words. The most dreadful words any person could hear. My Dad said, "Your great-grandmother died." I could hear his voice starting to crack and his eyes starting to fill with tears.

As he said these words, my heart completely stopped, my eyes started to gush with water like a hose, and my body started to fill with emotions of sadness. As I look around the room I see my mom's face bright red but not from anger, but from crying of sadness. My sister is huffing and puffing like the big bad wolf, and my dad, covering his face with his hands, is crying just slightly harder than the rest of us.

I sat on the couch, my eyes filling with tears and my vision starting to blur. I think back to the last good time I spent with my great-grandmother face to face.

"Ding Dong. Ding Dong." I heard as I rang the doorbell to go into my great-grandparent's house.

When I stepped inside their house, there was a cubby and a small little hallway, which led to the living room and a fresh smell in the air. I could see tons of my relatives, most of whom I usually see only in pictures. At that moment, I felt confused because I thought it was just us visiting. But soon my parents cleared my confusion and said that my other relatives wanted to see us all too. When I had fully walked into the room, I could see my great-grandmother sitting in her chair so lonely like a rock on the ground motionless. I felt so bad for her. Also, when I walked in, I'm blinded by the light going through the house.

We had to wheel my great-grandma to the table because it looked like she could not move. We sat down for dinner. The dinner table had been put in an awkward part of the room in the hallway.

"It is so delicious!" My grandma explained.

When we got up from dinner, they had to wheel my great-grandmother back to her chair's original spot.

"Earth to Madeline!" my dad shouts. That snapped me out of my trance back to reality!

"Yea I'm here," I replied.

I sit on my couch. I'm so lucky to have memories like these, I think to myself. I spend some time pondering how you never know when your last time will be with family.

~~~~~

In The Eyes of an Alzheimer's Patient
A letter from Kathleen Walsh

One day my dad, John C. Kuhn, was in our family home and he wanted to get something from the upstairs bedroom. Instead of heading up the stairs, he headed downstairs into the playroom area. The next thing I knew, I heard him pounding on the wall. My mom and I went running and he was hysterically crying and trying to explain that his mind was going. Over the next four years, we experienced the horrible disease called Alzheimer's.

My dad was an incredibly intelligent man. He served in WWII on the frontlines. He worked at IBM for thirty years. He was very involved in town politics. He studied to become a deacon in the Catholic Church at the age of seventy and was ordained and very proud. At the age of 74, his mind was not as sharp. He began to forget things like names and places. It caused him to get very angry because I think he knew what was happening.

I was the youngest of six children and definitely daddy's little girl. I also lived at home until marriage and then I made sure we lived close enough to see my parents daily. As the Alzheimer's progressed so did the anxiety and fear. I tried to help my mom after working all day. Band and I spent every weekend there, so mom could have a break. My dad started sleeping a lot during the day but would be up and about all night. Often, we would catch him packing suitcases, taking pictures off the walls, and trying to get out of the house.

Every day the deterioration would be a little worse. He could remember things from forty years ago like his first wife's passing, but he couldn't remember where he lived or what year it was. Our priest would come over at least once a week to pray with him and try to comfort him. My mom would hear him whispering, and later found out he was saying that mom, his wife of over thirty years, was trying to poison him. He would also see different things in our home that weren't there but you couldn't convince him otherwise. He saw snakes on the carpet and would pull his legs up in extreme fear. He thought everyone was trying to trick him or deceive him.

My brother was getting married during this ordeal and it was my job to take care of him and keep him safe so the wedding would be a success. They decided to have an evening reception which was typically his worst time. My firstborn was six weeks old so it was a busy time in my life. My father was so angry at the reception and he would tell anyone that would listen that he was packing up the house and moving. He would say that my mom, the kindest person, was evil and wanted him dead. He forgot who his family members were, but thankfully, he never forgot me. At the reception, I couldn't leave him alone. On the rare moments I had to, I would find him heading out the door or he would go back in the kitchen where food was being prepared. He did listen to me and I was able to steer him and reason sort of, but it was exhausting. Ten minutes later it would happen again.

My dad was also a very clean person with regard to hygiene and appearance. My husband used to say he dressed so well and looked like he came straight off a steam press. My mom did all of that for him. He was organized and particular. Then the disease progressed. He wouldn't shower and slowly stopped wanting to get dressed.

We took him to so many doctors and I honestly felt like they didn't listen or care. They spoke about characteristics, symptoms, and medication. I wanted to talk about my dad and I wanted a cure. I wanted them to cure it, and I wanted them to understand what our family was going through.

Each day would be a little worse than the day before. The next thing we knew, dad was in diapers and had lost all his dignity and respect. I constantly told him it would be OK and that he would get better. It would calm him.

Then he tried to get out of bed and fell. We took him to the hospital and it was almost as if he had a stroke. His mouth was wide open in a crooked way. I would walk in the room and he would say, "hi Kassabean," but with his mouth wide open. I was still thankful that he at least knew it was me. He couldn't eat, drink, or talk. My dear, sweet daddy didn't make it out of the hospital and passed away on August 1, 1994.

~~~~~~

A letter from Kaitlin Korcynski

My grandmother passed away from Alzheimer's 3 1/2 years ago. It was extremely difficult to watch her deteriorate.

My mother took on the task of sole caregiver as she lived closest to my grandma. It took a toll on our entire family, but mostly my mom. When my grandma was first diagnosed, my mom would be at her house multiple times a day making sure she was drinking enough water, eating three meals a day, getting out for walks, and taking care of her well-being. My mom was visiting with my grandma before work, during her lunch break, and after work each and every day. It was becoming a lot for my mom.

Unfortunately, as time progressed, so did my grandmother's Alzheimer's. In order to make things easier for our family and ensure my grandmother's health and safety, my mom and her siblings made the extremely difficult decision to move my grandmother into an assisted living facility. This was the best decision they could have made because it gave us many more years with my grandma, and made things easier for my mom. My mom continued to visit with my grandma every afternoon. I enjoyed being able to visit, too. My mom was especially grateful when I would tag along with her to visit. I was able to spend time and create more memories with my grandma and to provide support for my mom when things became difficult.

When she passed away, it was very difficult for us. We missed being able to spend time with her, hear her stories, and play games like Rummikub (her favorite). While trying to heal after her death, I came across this beautiful quote and it really stuck with me: "Memories are like sand castles - only by putting them in a safe place can you prevent them from washing away." I'm not sure who said this, but I am glad they did. Although my grandma had great difficulty with her memory, I know I can keep her memory and the memories we shared together safely in my heart - just like the many sand castles we used to build together at the beach.

Mrs. Damm was a very special person and I am so very lucky to have known her and been coached by you both! You always pushed us to be our best both in and out of the pool and I am a much better person because of it!

~~~~~

In The Eyes of an Alzheimer's Patient
A Letter From, Amber Mummert

Before, and early into the diagnosis, Grandma was a vibrant, sassy, quick-witted woman who loved running a tractor, splitting wood, sewing, crocheting, and cooking holiday meals for my large family. She and my grandfather, Arnold, were avid yard-sellers. They would scout out the paper for locations and go to as many as possible nearly every weekend in the spring and summer. I believe what she loved most of all, however, was supporting her grandkids at whatever extra-curricular activity they had and large family get-togethers. She had 5 kids, 13 grandchildren and I think 22 great-grandchildren at the time of her passing.

Grandma suffered through the disease for over a decade. First, forgetting where she just set her glass and repeating herself a little bit. Then names would slip her mind and she would forget what she had just done 5 minutes ago. After a while, she couldn't drive and couldn't be left alone. Then Grandpa had to unplug the stove so she wouldn't cook and leave burners on. Slowly she recognized fewer and fewer people and started telling the same story back-to-back. Eventually, she didn't know what foods she liked or disliked and would only like being around people on a "good day." She progressively got younger in her mind. Nearing the end, she could not dress or feed herself or go to the bathroom. Her words no longer were words, but rather the mumblings of an infant. Essentially, at the end of her life, she was a beautiful 83-year-old woman with the mind of a very young child.

The deterioration was difficult to watch for the entire family. However, it was definitely hardest on Grandpa. He was the one feeding her, medicating her, clipping her nails, bathing her, making sure she took her medicine, taking her to all her doctor's appointments, dressing her. He did EVERYTHING! He was her caretaker 24/7. Sometimes family would give him a break, but not nearly often enough. It's easy to see the strain it had on him, tired, sad, just worn out in general, but he kept on because she was the love of his life, and as he always said, "She would do the same for me."

~~~~~~

A Powerful Letter from Valerie Phillips, A Hospice Nurse

People say, "it must be so hard to be a hospice nurse. Bless you." Yes, of course, there are difficult moments, but the joy comes every day in providing care to a person who matters. Every person matters. I like to envision the world as a tapestry. Each of us is a colorful thread, weaving in and out of other peoples' lives. We never really know the potential of our connections. Hospice nursing is holistic – caring for the whole person – one connection at a time.

For the patient with Alzheimer's Disease, this understanding takes time; it takes collaboration with the caregiver. Every patient deserves to be given time and respect. This is not the "get in & get out," check-the-box kind of nursing. Who was this patient in the prime of their life? What values were important to them? What brought them simple joy? For Mary, it was completing a crossword puzzle, and by golly, she could still come up with answers to clues from some deep, untouched place in her brain.

Being a caregiver of a loved one with Alzheimer's can be exhausting and isolating. Quick trips to the grocery store, or time spent outdoors become a thing of the past. For decades, Mary and her spouse, Eugene, committed to long days at the pool coaching youth swimming. Shifting into caregiver role, Eugene was equally committed to doing what was right for Mary, from the hard work of maintaining skin integrity to respecting her requests for basic needs. This is full-time, 24/7, exhausting work for a caregiver. Even Eugene, who has a selfless personality, needed support in the home. He was appreciative when he found outside help who provided dignity to Mary, who in turn responded with compliance. Hospice care is a collaborative, providing support in the home with a team of clinical, social, personal, spiritual care experts, and let us not forget our invaluable volunteers. We empathize and work creatively to help the caregiver in their unique situation. Sometimes patients with Alzheimer's become verbally demanding; maybe we are simply support to the caregiver to say, yes, it's OK if the only thing they eat this week is chocolate ice cream.

Being a caregiver can also have beautiful, unexpected benefits. It can change your perspective on life; it can provide a purpose. If grandkids are around, they learn expressions of love through the actions of caregivers to their loved one with Alzheimer's. Maybe love is a daily leg rub with favorite lotion, maybe it's a project erecting a shower tent in the kitchen for the shower he always enjoyed. There are no regrets if caregivers truly connect with their loved one each day. As my friend Jules (LMSW), says, "We never know which day won't have a tomorrow." Even when people with Alzheimer's can no longer verbally communicate or seem absent, other senses can help connect – long, intentional eye contact if possible, stroking the hand, or humming a favorite tune or hymn.

No doubt as the disease progresses, the responsibilities and challenges to caregivers become fatiguing. Finding creative, individualized ways to help the caregiver keep the patient comfortable at home in a familiar environment brings me joy. It goes back to what I said earlier - every person has value in this tapestry of life, and I'll add, especially the caregivers.

Valerie V Phillips, BSN RN

~~~~~~

A Letter from Martha as a Companion and Caregiver

Caring for a person with Alzheimer's can be rewarding. Preparation before coming to their home or facility is helpful. Depending on their alertness will determine whether to interact with them or be passive in their care. Interaction includes conversation, playing cards, crossword puzzles, dominos, coloring, or Tic Tac Toe. Passive includes music, manicures, pedicures, lotion to arms and legs to help with relaxation.

The late afternoon, or early evening, tends to be when Sundowner's Syndrome affects a person with Alzheimer's. Instrumental music, turning off the television, and closing drapes help to calm them and helpsthem sleep at night.

Being flexible helps. Some activity that doesn't help, try another activity.

~~~~~~

In The Eyes of an Alzheimer's Patient

A Note From the Author

I talk to my wife as I look at her picture of her final years of happiness. It is the picture that now hangs on our bedroom wall. It was enlarged and placed next to her casket at the funeral ceremony. It is in this book for a reason. It portrays her with her Cape Cod sweatshirt, holding both our ice cream cones. Both the place and ice cream were dear to her. It shows her happy in her later years before the tragedy of Alzheimer's. Despite being an extrovert, she very seldom posed with a smile. In this picture, as well as some other chosen pictures, you certainly can imagine the joy in her heart when she was in her "element."

Talking to her might sound eccentric, but many a spouse of a deceased person has engaged in similar experiences in this type of communication. This helps to remember the good times together. It is the strength of the bond between two married people that shapes their life together. As you have seen, we melded our characters to be one. We did this through our marriage and in our long career as swimming coaches while balancing work, family, and other volunteering, as well as our religious life.

Mary co-authored our swimming books and she was the inspiration that caused me to write this book. I wrote a lot about my career in the early chapters as it is important to know how a man who was in charge of a number of things in his work life, became submissive in just about everything to take care of his wife. The change in the caregiver's life is especially dramatic, particularly if the afflicted spouse did many of the household chores as Mary did for our family. It was the old-fashioned way and I eventually had to learn how to do things that were foreign to me under very adverse conditions. Keep in mind that it is not me in the specific, it is really an illustration of what a profound change can take place in the life of any caregiver. There are people who experience tougher conditions than I did, as they strive to prevent the patient from doing anything that would be injurious to themselves. I shudder to think how people have to worry about keeping the exterior doors locked, the car keys hidden, and the stove guarded, among a host of other things on their mind.

It is important to keep in mind how a relatively poor boy with an inferiority complex, struggled in making friends and had a tendency to be a follower would overcome these attributes through the help of his wife. Any success I had was as much of a success for her as it was for me. She prompted me to do many things which changed my own life to a more meaningful one. It would not have happened without her. The change from someone whose wife shopped and cooked for him, as well as doing all the household tasks and bringing up our children, was as dramatic a change as it could be, but the mental turmoil was worse. The man who rarely changed a diaper for his children was now attending to an adult.

Again, throughout this book, keep in mind that we are only examples of many people who are experiencing, or will experience, extreme changes in their life as they take care of their loved one with Alzheimer's. This cannot be stressed enough by our own examples in this book. Alzheimer's disease attacks people of every status in life. It can attack presidents and multi-millionaires, as well as low-income people. It is the disease that captures your mind, which then insidiously attacks your body. There is no escape regardless of your financial status, or your fame as an outstanding medical professional, artist, or author.

In The Eyes of an Alzheimer's Patient

It is interesting that the people who knew us from our later activities, knew us as the team of Gene and Mary, but as the reader will see in our personal life it was the team of Mary and Gene. It was she who encouraged me to follow only one career, as my health deteriorated. It was Mary who let me continue to coach after a very serious health issue. It was she who convinced me to go back to volunteer coaching after we retired from college coaching in the profession I came to love. Mary continued to encourage me to do more than I was doing, even when she reached the level that she needed more care. It was her always wanting to make me happy doing the things I enjoyed.

While this book seems to portray life and a near-perfect marriage, it does not portray a number of the disagreements and confrontations, some more serious than others, that can occur in married life and certainly occurred with us. However, they are inconsequential and of short term in the scope of the life of two people bonded together as tightly as we were. We were truly a team in everything. In Mary's spiritual authorship, she talked about the wall of happiness built up in our lives, and how the crumbling of it did not alter the fact that we were two people who became one on our wedding day. We meshed perfectly in the things that mattered most for our happiness. This is the story of our life before, and after Mary's affliction with the dreaded Alzheimer's disease. It involves both her as a victim and me as her caregiver. But it could be any two people. Except for what I believe could be going on in the mind of the patient, this story is as true as I can make it, even my shortcomings. I felt it was more powerful to portray real characters than write a totally fictional novel.

The beginning of the story outlined our early lives and our rise to a higher status. It will seem to be boasting in parts about me as the person who had two responsible jobs and carried them out successfully. I feel the boasting helps the reader realize that Mary, in changing my personality, had a large role in my ability to reach whatever achievements I had, especially in my coaching. She was essential in just about everything we did. Also, it shows that, regardless of success and happiness, Alzheimer's changes the life of anyone, be they a caregiver or a patient.

I loved to teach in everything I did, both in industry and coaching. But a teaching degree option was not open to me as a career. With my subdued personality and my inferiority complex at the time, I was not sure that I could do the job right anyway.

God blessed me with Mary, who helped bring me out of my shell and to bring me to my real teaching avocation; a career helping youngsters up to college-age swimmers and beyond. Mary was the vehicle to get me started in helping young people, and in urging me to continue even after she encountered Alzheimer's. I also enjoyed my career with IBM, but I enjoyed coaching more. The stories I boasted of are true, to the extent I can make them, and they powerfully demonstrate that people, no matter how high and mighty they become, can be seriously degraded by the incurable disease called Alzheimer's. It doesn't just take your life, it also degrades you to the lowest level of mankind.

There is a picture that one of my lesson swimmer's family gave me when their boy left for college. It still hangs near the front door of our house. I can only hope that it exemplifies our life of interacting with the many swimmers, up through college age, that were under our guidance. The text from that picture embodies the importance and honor achieved from working with youth.

One Hundred Years from now
It will not matter
what kind of car I drove,
what kind of house I lived in,
how much money was in my bank account
nor what my clothes looked like.
But the world may be a better place because
I was important in the life of a child.[2]

In The Eyes of an Alzheimer's Patient

I wrote the story as if Mary, the diseased Alzheimer's patient, were recalling her life and the life of her husband, the caregiver. Mary and I are true-life people, used as examples, and our story describes how we were impacted by this dreadful disease. The description of what occurred in the mind of Mary is from my perspective and are in a sense fictional, but I hope the portrayal of her many thoughts fairly describes our existence in helping others. The stories are real, but hopefully, the reader can relate to their own lives as they read this book, and then put Alzheimer's into the equation, to realize the massive impact it would or could have on them.

There were minor, and sometimes major falls from the steep wall of happiness that formed our lives, but we always recouped like the phoenix of mythology rising from the ashes. That is until Alzheimer's came into our lives. The disease is insidious and not always recognized, especially in people who start out at a higher state of intelligence and are of advanced age. It is more common in the elderly. However, it can also assail people of a younger age, as it did for a friend of ours. He was in his early 40's when he passed away. It is like slow-moving lava coming down from an erupting volcano, and you are immobile, not able to get away from it. For older people, the early stages may look like some type of aging cognitive recognition problem, where you are worse than usual at remembering recent events. Later, it may seem that you are experiencing some form of mild dementia. A casual look by a physician may have it called vascular dementia at some stage. However, as the stages progress, they may suggest seeing a neurologist for testing, which is really when the disease can be diagnosed.

Alzheimer's can be looked at as an extreme version of dementia, and I mean extreme. At even later stages, one may not be able to remember family and friends. It is difficult for the ones you love to see your mind die and then see your bodily functions deteriorate. Anger seems to be the outlet a patient uses when they cannot answer a question. They then panic as a result of frustrations when they experience difficulty in making things happen.

Eventually, one may not be able to walk, drink, or eat, as their mind seems to break down the bodily functions, and they are not able to control them. They may want to roam around outside at night, or remove their clothes, especially if the clothing feels "too tight" for reasons unknown. When the end comes, you would think that it would at least be peaceful for the patient suffering from the blitzkrieg of Alzheimer's. However, although that may be true, it is not always a consolation to those who remember you as you once were. Your mouth may be open in a distorted way. This can be common in the later stages of Alzheimer's, a horrible reminder of the destructive force of this disease. Those that see you in that state may feel the pangs of remorse for the suffering that was endured, as you left this life in a state which was not you.

The picture before them is not a pretty one. It is also not just the death that they will remember, but the dramatic changes in your life. It is not the "you," that they would like to remember. Embalming does not totally bring back the picture of you, but you look better than with your mouth distorted as if you were in true agony. Those that only see you there at rest and in peace, do not realize the earlier picture that your family had to sadly experience.

The early to mid-stages of this book showed a life that may seem like the setting of a goody-goody movie, even as the book progresses, to the point where Alzheimer's rears its ugly head. But the events are not part of a movie. They are real. I did have two careers for much of my working life. Mary did also for a shorter while. We were still able to balance our lives because Mary was a significant figure in our second careers as swimming coaches. Mary not only managed the house but also brought up the children and cared for a sick mother and father. Coaching took significant time out of our personal lives, but we still managed it without much sacrifice of what we considered our duties.

We coached together, starting out as volunteers, and then eventually as paid coaches. Most coaches do not have the advantage of being a husband and wife team. Swimming meets, especially those of three or more days including preliminary events for all age groups that were followed by finals for the senior swimmers, allowed little time for us to recuperate. The impact on coaches being away from their spouses for these events could have a detrimental effect on their married life.

Coaching together, and with our children being swimmers in the early ages, made it easier for us. But you will see some of the health issues that endangered both Mary and my life as a result of this lifestyle. We considered these issues as bumps in the road which would not stop us from helping younger, and college-age swimmers, grow into mature and responsible adults. The fact that we produced swimmers at the national level was not the only important thing in life. We hoped that we also served as role models in the development of our swimmers as mature adults. Only our former swimmers can attest to that. To understand us a little better, you have to know, on weekend meets and training trips, we never missed Sunday Mass, regardless of where we were in the country.

We were really a team in much of our efforts, as you've seen, as our story unfolds. As far as I am concerned, we are still a team. I look at Mary's picture and she spiritually guides me, even though she is not physically here. She inspires me to do things, such as writing this book. I knew some of her inner thoughts better than anybody, and while these thoughts may seem fictional to some, they may be real in the eyes of many Alzheimer's patients.

I had a somewhat unique personality, in that when I had to lead, I could and would take charge when no one else did. When everything was going well, I could be totally subordinate, and willingly let others take charge, as long as the job was done right. Whatever my job, and regardless of the pay, I would give my all. That was also apparent with both of us in our married life, and certainly when we were swimming coaches.

Mary managed the money, pushed me to take vacations, and to take rest stops on long trips. She even picked out my clothes. It was the perfect relationship for her and me. I was a workaholic and she was the tempering entity to try to keep me from hurting myself, more than I did. I had some life-endangering experiences, probably from overwork as a result of my two jobs, but they might have been worse, or have come earlier in life, had she not been there.

She was responsible for morphing me from a subdued quiet young boy, to a man who could handle himself in today's world. I, in turn, took a young girl and gave her a reason to live for another person. I depended on her to not only watch over our house and family but to be a motivator and supportive co-worker in our service efforts. We were a perfect match. As they say, it was a marriage made in Heaven. The ups and downs were minuscule compared to the pleasures we had together in our efforts to help children become responsible adults, using swimming as the impetus.

This book is also intended to show the reality of the quote, that "love is stronger than death," and remains a theme throughout this book. I normally like to have a shock in my mystery novels that surprises the reader, but there are no shocks, only the inevitable, with this disease. The only shock is with the reactions of the patient's loved ones. Even though everyone knows the end is near, the shock can only be realized by the persons experiencing the death of a loved one, especially with Alzheimer's. I myself did not realize that Mary's death would leave such an enduring impact, even on our great-grandchildren. But it did, and it still does.

While this is our story, it could also be any two people in any walk of life. Beggars and kings in this world share the same illnesses, with the resulting agony, for them and others who care for them. We are only one example in the middle.

In The Eyes of an Alzheimer's Patient

I leave this portion of the book with the aforementioned quote. I hope that you will excuse the boasts, but they are relevant to reinforcing that success does not protect one from this disease. With that important message, always remember that:

"Love is stronger than death"

Gene Damm

A Few Words about Alzheimer's

Alzheimer's disease is named after doctor Alois Alzheimer who studied the brain tissue of a patient (Frau Auguste Deter) with presenile, along with unpredictable, behavior. Frau Deter was a woman of only 51, who was brought to the Institution for the Mentally Ill when her husband felt that he was no longer able to control her odd behavior. Doctor Alzheimer originally diagnosed her with presenile dementia but was fascinated by her condition at such a relatively early age. She had severe short-term memory issues and could not remember objects shortly after they were presented to her. When asked her name, she would answer "Auguste," but when asked her husband's name, she would again answer with her name. When she was eating and asked what it was, she said "spinach" when actually it was pork. At night things worsened, her speech was confusing and she would wake up screaming. She stayed at the institute for five years and passed away in 1906. Doctor Alzheimer, who was at the Royal Psychiatric Clinic in Munich, requested that her brain and medical records be sent to him so he could analyze them. He discovered atrophy of the part of the brain that is responsible for language, judgment, and thought. Although Frau Deter had Alzheimer's at an early age, it was a benchmark study named in 1910 after the first person to study it so deeply.[3] Keep in mind that in over 100 years no one has been able to find a way to separate Alzheimer's from other symptoms of old age or simple dementia in the early stages without professional testing. Nor has there been an effective and affordable medicine to significantly slow down or put Alzheimer's into full remission.

It was only until fairly recent years that people with mental challenges such as severe Alzheimer's were sent to what was called insane asylums. There, they would be patients, sometimes constrained in straitjackets and/or placed in padded cells. There are horror stories on the Internet of some of the physical abuse of patients at specific asylums. Some even performed a lobotomy with an ice pick. My father worked at a New Jersey institution for a short time and told us one story of patient abuse. I am sure there were also good stories in many of the institutions, but as usual, we do not normally hear of them. Most of these asylums eventually closed due to the shift in medical treatments and public perception, as well as financial instability. Unfortunately, the massive closing of asylums was considered a failure as it was not well thought out concerning the transition to self-reliance even when on medication. There apparently were not enough educated caregivers and the availability of other medical facilities to adequately take care of the patients. If one does not have insurance and there is no institution left with a primary goal to take care of Alzheimer's patients, the burden falls on the family, if they can manage it.

Alzheimer's is one of the most wicked forms of the broad categories called dementia. It starts out mildly, then increases steadily until it captures all one's critical functions. One essentially dissolves into a death spiral as the brain impairs one's ability to survive. The Mayo Clinic reported that 5.8 million people in the United States age 65 and older live with Alzheimer's disease.[4] Although the death rate is high, it can actually be much higher depending on how the data are recorded. Many people with Alzheimer's usually have other health issues that can lead to early death. Alzheimer's accelerates these issues, thus robbing them of their natural responses to nourish their body and survive. While it may not be the direct cause of death, Alzheimer's can cause problems that lead the patient to a stage where other life-threatening issues, such as heart failure, accelerate to early death. The number of deaths attributed to Alzheimer's between 2000 and 2019 has more than doubled. Also, one in three seniors dies from Alzheimer's or other dementia according to the Alzheimer's Association.[5]

Caring for a loved one with Alzheimer's can also be devastating for the caregiver. One source stated that approximately 70% of Alzheimer's patients exhibit some type of aggression.[6] This aggression, combined with symptoms of agitation, can take its toll on the caregiver who has to deal with it. Medicines to control aggression have to be strictly controlled by a doctor, as they can lead to other complications including early death in elderly patients.

Understanding the inheritance of Alzheimer's is difficult. As an example, there is a rare mutation of genes that show up in a small number of families that seem to catalyze the onset of Alzheimer's disease at an early age.[7] More work needs to be done here.

There is a common variant of a gene that increases one's life-long risk of Alzheimer's which can be tested for by genetic analysis. However, there are people who can carry this gene and may not be affected by it. At the moment, it is considered only as a risk factor. Since there presently are no good treatments to halt the progression of the disease, unless you have a history of Alzheimer's in your family, there is little to gain by testing.

Risk factors only point to the fact that one may be subject to a health problem, but there is no guarantee that it will happen if one leads a healthy lifestyle. Leading a healthy lifestyle with exercise, proper nutrition, and maintaining a proper body mass index (BMI) may even have a greater impact than anything else at the moment to prevent and slow down Alzheimer's.[8] Without a cure, a healthy lifestyle may be the only weapon against the disease. The Federal Government needs to spend more money on Alzheimer's research with grants, especially to small companies specializing in this area. Funding is needed for research into the causes of Alzheimer's plus diagnostic tests for the disease. This information will assist research into treatments where funding is also needed.

Recently, the Federal Drug Administration (FDA) approved Aduhelm, developed by Biogen, as the first drug considered a "disease-modifying" therapy for Alzheimer's.[9] It was designed to remove tiny deposits in the brains called amyloid plaques. These were first described by Dr. Alzheimer after examining sections of Frau Deter's brain under a microscope.[3] It has been exciting news that a new therapy can remove these plaques that are often considered diagnostic for Alzheimer's disease, but unfortunately, the evidence that Aduhelm can also improve cognition is much less clear, and the drug is both expensive and carries safety risks.

Developing new drugs that can have an effect on improving cognition is not an easy task. It is much like the crow in an Aesop fable, who was thirsty and wanted to drink the water he saw in the bottom of a jug, but the neck was too narrow to drink from. He came up with the idea of dropping pebbles in the jug until the water reached the top, much like if you filled a pot of water for soup then tried to put too many ingredients in it and the water spilled over the stove. We may need a lot of pebbles in the jug of knowledge before we can drink of the curing water to halt dementia, and more specifically Alzheimer's in vulnerable people. And I might add that the research done to produce new drugs can be horrendous and there are not many companies that can afford the upfront cost, never mind the ability to recoup the development cost.

Some publications talk about having seven stages of Alzheimer's.[1] Others sort them in only three stages, such as mild, moderate, and severe. I showed the seven stages at the beginning of this book for academic purposes. To the caregivers, all they see is simply a transition from one agonizing phase to another. The attack on certain brain functions may produce many similar reactions, but sometimes different reactions may manifest themselves in particular patients. One patient may know who their spouse of many years is, but believe that they are trying to do something to poison them. Others may seemingly recognize their spouse as the person they love, but not other friends or family members, as yet another example.

To better understand the disease, let's compare it in retrograde. Think of the development of a child. First, there are unintelligible sounds, then gradually one begins to understand the jargon. Then the child finally reaches the stage of full communication. Alzheimer's is the reverse of that description. In the case of the child developing, you have joy and look forward to the next change. In the case of the Alzheimer's patient, you have sadness and frustration, and wish the next change would never come, or at least would take longer to develop.

Currently, there is no cure for Alzheimer's. There is only an agonizing progression. There is no Praetorian Guard in your mind to protect you once it has infiltrated. People ask me "When did Mary's Alzheimer's start?" or "How long did she have it?" The answer is always the same... I don't know. Neither did the doctors know who treated her. One of our primary doctors told her in a somewhat happy voice that she had vascular dementia. They said it was not Alzheimer's when it was mentioned. He may not have been terribly wrong in that diagnosis because of the stage she was at, but it points out that you cannot tell the difference many times until you perform a series of tests as Alzheimer's progresses.

To truly understand a disease, you have to know how it was built in order to dismantle it, and even that may be a difficult task. Building a puzzle may be difficult, but dismantling it is easy. Once you have built a puzzle and dismantled it you know the clues, and the puzzle is much less challenging. Alzheimer's still needs to be understood better, like a number of diseases, to effectively destroy it. There needs to be as much research on Alzheimer's as there is for other diseases with a similar death rate. The disease is insidious and the temptation in the early stages is to say, "old age is creeping up" and it is a natural progression within the life cycle. Think about all the jokes made about older people's forgetfulness. Like in our story, the hospital staff tried to convince my family that the symptoms I was having were attributable to old age when in reality I really had a severe brain bleed that needed immediate attention. When even some medical professionals look at old age as the only reason for odd behavior in the elderly, you know how common and tempting it is to soothe family members with that rationale.

With people living longer and recognizing that this disease attacks the elderly at a higher rate, we do need to recognize it in as early a stage as possible. Recognition can be done by means of available testing, if for no other reason than to alert the family members as to what they are up against. Even more importantly, we need to find a cure. A cure that at least makes Alzheimer's dormant for a while before the death rate becomes more intolerable by ending life too early, even if there were no immediate signs of other life-ending illnesses.

Let's take a look at a commonly used tool, a claw hammer perfectly matched for you. It may seem simple to build after you know what is needed. What may appear simple, though, is not always the case. To build a perfect claw hammer for yourself, you would have to understand the perfect weight for the job and balance that against your own strength. The length, shape, and width of the handle would be determined by these factors along with the roll of the wrist in providing maximum efficiency. The length, width, and shape of the claw would have to be calculated for maximum leverage. It's not so simple.

Now let's graduate to all the physics required that our mind has to go through to ride a bicycle. It is not quite as simple as you would think, but in building the features, your mind can test them out and do all the work rather than you having to make a number of mathematical computations. Now measure that mathematical complexity a thousand times, or more, and you may understand the complexity for scientists to understand the complete chemistry of a disease like Alzheimer's. Even understanding it, the testing that would be needed to prove the efficacy of the therapeutic solution in most cases is a long and arduous task.

The above examples are lessons in how your mind easily solves what would be usually a physics problem to control a robot. It should get you thinking about the fact that your mind is working at 100 percent to produce an efficient solution. But what if it is only working at 25 or less percent. That is what is happening in the later stages of Alzheimer's.

For many other horrible diseases, we have been able to produce a cure, or at least have the ability to produce a benign state for an extended period of time. We are not there yet with Alzheimer's disease. We may be able to slow down the disease somewhat at times with medicine, but we cannot stop the progress. The disease can attack people who are seemingly well. No other disease or weakness may be apparent, or there may be other issues such as diabetes and heart issues that consume the patient and their family, while Alzheimer's is doing its heinous job. Alzheimer's can attack the brain so slowly, that it is not recognized until it overcomes thought processes enough that the patient's odd behavior becomes noticeable. Even then, in elderly people, it can look like simple dementia. That is bad enough, but it continues to attack the brain until the person you knew and loved is unrecognizable as they become a body with less and less brain function.

Mary lost most of her brain function to a great degree, but surprisingly enough could be a whiz working with someone to verbally solve crossword puzzles, almost to the end of life. Martha, the caregiver, who was sent to give me respite, and cared for Mary, will tell you that you have to keep patiently working to find something they enjoy doing with a hidden part of their brain still alive and functioning. Valerie, the treasured hospice nurse who was in charge of Mary's home care, also emphasized this. The patient may not know the year, recognize some family members, or even you, but if you search hard enough, you will probably be able to give Alzheimer's a run for its money.

Alzheimer's affects the mind, and the mind affects bodily functions. The death certificate may read that the primary cause of death is perhaps a failure of the heart or some other bodily function, but if you lose your ability to recognize hunger or thirst, and are in a weak state, unable to breathe properly, the real villain may be Alzheimer's. Providing more oxygen in the absence of food and drink to the body will not stop the mind of the patient from having an automatic death spiral response, which makes death inevitable.

That is when it is difficult determining the actual cause of death, especially when other factors are present. If the patient's heart is weak, the death certificate may read that the cause of death was heart failure, with Alzheimer's, diabetes, etc. listed as ancillary diseases. But if the patient is not able to eat or drink, and even medication has to be given by syringe with massaging of the cheek to induce swallowing, then how can the bodily functions do their job? What is the real cause of death? When the heart fails, the question is what role did Alzheimer's play in setting conditions where the heart could not properly operate?

Some interesting statistics published by the Alzheimer's Association include the fact that approximately five million Americans are living with this disease, and every 66 seconds a new person in the United States develops it.[5] A couple of other interesting statistics are that Alzheimer's Disease kills more people than breast cancer, prostate cancer, and hypertension combined. Since 2000, deaths by heart disease have decreased by approximately 14 percent while Alzheimer's disease and other dementia deaths have increased by approximately 89 percent. It is the sixth leading cause of death in the United States and it is the only one in the top 10 which cannot be prevented, cured, or slowed down to any great extent. Certain medications may temporarily slow down the progression, but there is no cure. These statistics show that much more work needs to be done to determine how we can defeat Alzheimer's.

Since my wife Mary has passed, I am a vehicle to share what goes on in the mind of an Alzheimer's patient, as they undergo the transition from an active life to one of vagaries and total dependence on a caregiver. Many caregivers are spouses, who, because of the physical and mental strain on them, pass away before the patient. Sad statistic, but true.

This situation may have caused some serious health challenges for me. I had already suffered some health issues caused by stress in trying to do two jobs to the best of my ability. I was working for IBM and pursuing our swimming coaching careers at the same time. The coaching job sometimes took seven days a week in preparation for weekend meets. But Mary and I did it together, and that made it acceptable. The stress of working and doing something you love is nothing compared to the 24/7 care of a loved one with Alzheimer's. Your health can deteriorate faster than you realize if you do not have any time to reduce stress.

When I was coaching after a hard day at IBM, I could totally focus on my coaching, which I enjoyed, to relieve the stress. The role of a 24/7 caregiver does not allow that luxury without the assistance and support of professional caregivers. Very few are free, so the full advantage of a professional caregiver may be out of range for many families. If they search hard enough, though, they may find state agencies that offer free respite services. In addition, the Alzheimer's Association and a number of other agencies and societies including the Mayo Clinic can provide useful information. However, there are not many options for taking away the evening stress of caring for an Alzheimer's patient who is having a troubling night.

In this book, I focus on myself as the caregiver to serve as a warning to future caregivers that they may have life-threatening issues if they reject respite help as I did at times. You must always remember that you have to be alive and well to take care of your loved one.

There may not be a cure now for Alzheimer's. Early death is inevitable, but remember that it is not only the patient that is impacted by this disease. The lifespan and quality of life of the caregiver can also be impaired just when the loved one needs them by their side the most.

Gene Damm

Acknowledgments

My thanks to the people who donated letters and photographs and to my family who not only provided me with the letters in the book but also gave me advice on improving it. A special thanks to Tom Morris who helped in the initial formatting, and has been a great help in this, and past books, as well as Clark Bullock and Pamela Warner who graciously agreed to review the book. I cannot leave out my publisher Robin Nelson and her husband Bob. Bob gave me a tutorial on the role of specific genes that have been looked at for their potential role in Alzheimer's. I hope that I got it right. Nor can I forget Elaine Forgue, from the New Bedford High School staff, who days before her retirement, diligently looked through and photographed a number of class book photographs for possible use in this book and others who provided photographs to use. Lastly, let me give a special thanks to Brian Tutko who did the final editing,

Resources

1. The Alzheimer's Association has a 24/7 helpline and local support groups, along with being a valuable source of information on Alzheimer's. (866-232-8484)(https://alzfdn.org/)

2. The Alzheimer's Foundation of America (AFA) has a help line and offers support for caregivers and for people diagnosed with Alzheimer's. (http://alzfdn.org/)

3. Elder care locator can connect the caregiver with local resources and support groups. for support and training of the caregiver, (https://eldercare.acl.gov/Public/Index.aspx)

4. Family Caregiver Alliance is where online the caregiver can discuss their challenges, concerns, and rewards. (https://www.caregiver.org/)

5. Memory People is a facebook page where a person can find information and share experiences as a caregiver. (https://www.facebook.com/Memory-People-126017237474382/)

6. The Veteran's Administration Caregiver Support Line is a toll-free number for caregivers, family members, friends, Veterans, and community partners to contact for information related to caregiving and available supports and services. (1-855-260-3274).

References

1. Barry Reisberg, M.D, retrieved (December 7, 2021) *Clinical Stages of Alzheimer's*, https://www.alzwa.org/files/2015/01/07-Clinical-Stages-of-Alzheimer.pdf

2. Witcraft, Forest, *Within My Power*, October, Scouting Magazine,1950.

3. Alzheimer's Association, https://www.alz.org/alzheimers-dementia/research_progress/milestones.

4. The Mayo Clinic, (https://www.mayoclinic.org/diseases-conditions/alzheimers-disease/symptoms-causes/syc-20350447)

5. The Alzheimer's Organization, https://www.alz.org/alzheimers-dementia/facts-figures#:~:text=Alzheimer's%20kills.,Alzheimer's%20disease%20have%20increased%20significantly.

6. Ballard, Clive; Corbett, Anne, Current Opinion in Psychiatry, 26(3):252-259, May 2013.

7. NIH, https://www.nia.nih.gov/health/what-causes-alzheimers-disease

8. Mayo Clinic, https://www.mayoclinic.org/diseases-conditions/alzheimers-disease/symptoms-causes/syc-20350447

9. WebMD, https://www.webmd.com/alzheimers/aduhelm-what-to-know

Other Books by Gene Damm

Swimming Books for Charity by Gene Damm with Mary Damm:

- *Guide for Competitive Swimmers*
- *Fast Swimming with Mind over Water*
- *Fast Swimming with Technique and Mental Awareness*

Mystery Books for Charity by Gene Damm:

- *Death Took a Dive*
- *Accident or Murder*
- *Where Are the Kids*

Gene Damm

Lightning Source UK Ltd.
Milton Keynes UK
UKHW020833270223
417728UK00016B/1366